Questions and Answers for Diploma in Dental Nursing, Level 3

Questions and Answers for Diploma in Dental Nursing, Level 3

Carole Hollins

General Dental Practitioner
Member of the British Dental Association
Former Chairman and Presiding Examiner for the National Examining Board for Dental Nurses

WILEY Blackwell

Library of Congress Cataloging-in-Publication Data

Hollins, Carole, author.
  Questions and answers for Diploma in dental nursing, level 3 / Carole Hollins.
     p. ; cm.
  Complemented by: Diploma in dental nursing, level 3 / Carole Hollins. Third edition. 2014.
  Includes index.
  ISBN 978-1-118-92378-8 (pbk.)
I. Hollins, Carole. Diploma in dental nursing, level 3. Complemented by (work):   II. Title.
[DNLM: 1. Dental Assistants–Examination Questions.   2. Dental Care–methods–Examination Questions.   WU 18.2]
  RK60.5
  617.6'0233076–dc23
                                                2015006396
A catalogue record for this book is available from the British Library.

Set in 9.5/13pt Meridien by SPi Global, Pondicherry, India
Printed and bound by CPI Group (UK) Ltd, Croydon, CR0 4YY

C9781118923788_140224

Contents

Introduction

The vast majority of dental nurses in the United Kingdom currently achieve registerable qualification and regulation by the General Dental Council by one of two routes: the City & Guilds Diploma in Dental Nursing, Level 3, or the National Examining Board for Dental Nurses' National Diploma. Although the same qualification is awarded to successful candidates following either route to registration, the training and assessment methods involved for each are quite different.

In recent years the assessment methods in particular for each qualification have diverged, and it has become prudent to provide separate revision aids for each group of students. This book is aimed at those studying for the City & Guilds Diploma in Dental Nursing, Level 3. A companion textbook is available (*Diploma in Dental Nursing, Level 3*, third edition), and a separate textbook and revision aid are also available for those following the National Diploma route to qualification (*Levison's Textbook for Dental Nurses*, eleventh edition, *Questions & Answers for Dental Nurses*, third edition).

This new book is set out with relevant questions which cover every assessment criteria of the Level 3 Diploma curriculum, laid out in Units 312, 313, 314 and 315. These four units provide the theory and underpinning knowledge on which the students' written examination paper is based, while other parts of the curriculum are assessed by observation in the dental workplace. Students must complete both the necessary observation portfolio and pass the written paper before being awarded their registerable qualification.

The book layout follows that used successfully for the past 18 years for National Diploma (previously National Certificate) students, in that explanatory notes following the correct answer for each question are included in an effort to help explain not just why one answer option is correct, but often more importantly why the other options are incorrect. Students have found this additional information, often explained in an alternative manner to that used in the textbook, as highly useful in providing a greater depth of knowledge to a subject.

It is hoped that all students using this book will find it both instructive and informative, and an invaluable revision aid in their quest for qualification.

Happy reading to all.

How to Use This book

Diploma in Dental Nursing, Level 3 curriculum covers 15 units as set out in the companion textbook *Diploma in Dental Nursing, Level 3*, third edition. The first 11 units are assessed by observation in the workplace (or an appropriate alternative method), while the last four units are assessed by a written examination paper containing multiple-choice and short-answer questions. This book has been written as a revision aid for students studying for this qualification, by providing suitably styled questions covering all of the learning outcomes in these four units. More importantly, the correct answer to each question is also provided and with an accompanying explanation so that students can maximise their learning at every opportunity.

The four units which provide the theory and underpinning knowledge on which the questions have been based are as follows:

- Unit 312 – Principles of infection control in the dental environment
- Unit 313 – Assessment of oral health and treatment planning
- Unit 314 – Dental radiography
- Unit 315 – Scientific principles in the management of oral health diseases and dental procedures

Each of the units is divided in the curriculum into a varying number of learning outcomes, and these are further subdivided into assessment criteria for each outcome – it is these assessment criteria that provide the basis for the questions.

The book is laid out with a chapter for each learning outcome, and the questions are set randomly to cover all of the associated assessment criteria for that chapter. The second part of each chapter contains the correct answers given in the same order as the questions, and with explanatory notes to help students better understand the relevant theory if they find their own answers are incorrect.

So as an example, Chapter 1 relates to Unit 312, learning outcome 1 which states 'understand the process of infection control'. The 25 questions the chapter contains then randomly cover the three assessment criteria associated with this outcome:

1 Describe the causes of cross-infection.
2 Describe the methods for preventing cross-infection.
3 Explain the principles of standard (universal) infection control precautions.

Obviously then, more than one question has been set for each assessment criteria.

Each question is set as a question stem followed by four possible answers: A, B, C or D. Only one option will be correct for each question. To encourage students to determine a correct answer by logic rather than by guessing, and in line with best educational practice, the answers are always set out alphabetically or numerically in ascending order rather than randomly. This removes the element of, say, choosing answer B because the previous answer was not B, and so on.

Throughout the book, there are several questions which ask the student to choose an answer which is either a true statement or a false statement, and great care must be taken to ensure that the question stem has been read correctly and that all four options are read fully before answering. It is very easy to choose what is thought to be a valid answer early on at option A and miss determining a more suitable answer at option C or D – this style of question requires the student to have both appropriate knowledge and effective reasoning skills to be completed correctly.

An example of this question style is shown below.

Which one of the following statements regarding the clinical hand-washing technique is false:

A Antibacterial soap should be used
B Illustrated directions should be present at each hand-washing sink
C Rinsing should occur towards the fingers
D Taps should not be hand-operated

Finally, although the questions are based around the final four units of the qualification curriculum, students will realise during their studies that the unit contents also link back to various of the other 11 units. So the theory and underpinning knowledge covered in Unit 312 links back to information covered in Unit 301 (ensure your own actions reduce risks to health and safety) and Unit 304 (prepare and maintain environment, instruments and equipment for clinical dental procedures). The student is therefore encouraged to begin using this revision aid as soon as possible during their studies, rather than just in the run up to sitting the written examination paper, in the hope that they gain the maximum benefit from its content, and that it provides the optimum learning opportunities for their studies.

UNIT 312

Principles of Infection Control in the Dental Environment

OUTCOME 1

Understand the Process of Infection Control

Questions

1 Hand hygiene is important in minimising the risk of cross infection in the dental workplace. Which one of the following levels of hand hygiene aims to physically remove routinely acquired microorganisms?

   A Clinical

   B Hygienic

   C Social

   D Surgical

2 Cross infection may occur in the dental workplace in a variety of ways. Which one of the following options describes the least likely method for a cross-infection incident to occur in a well-organised environment?

   A Aerosol spray

   B Direct contact

   C Inoculation injury

   D Particle spatter

3 What is the correct term used to describe a person who is infected with a pathogenic microorganism but who shows no outward signs of disease?

   A Carrier

   B Contaminated

   C High risk

   D Infectious

Questions and Answers for Diploma in Dental Nursing, Level 3, First Edition. Carole Hollins.
© 2016 John Wiley & Sons, Ltd. Published 2016 by John Wiley & Sons, Ltd.

4 There are various levels of cleanliness referred to in the clinical setting. Which one of the following options is the term used when only bacteria and fungi have been destroyed by the cleaning method involved?

  A Aseptic

  B Disinfected

  C Socially clean

  D Sterilised

5 Various methods are used in the dental workplace to prevent cross-infection incidents. Which one of the following options is the term used to describe the method of removing potential aerosol and droplet contamination between dental procedures?

  A Barrier method

  B Surface cleaning

  C Use of disposables

  D Zoning

6 Which one of the following is an example of a potential indirect cross-infection incident?

  A Clean inoculation injury

  B Use of disinfected extraction forceps

  C Use of a disposable aspirator tip

  D Use of a new endodontic hand file

7 There are various methods available to the dental team for preventing cross infection in the dental workplace. Which one of the following options is the most effective method of preventing cross infection between patients?

  A Use of autoclave

  B Use of barrier methods

  C Use of disposable items

  D Use of washer–disinfector

8 While working in the dental workplace, the dental team will always try to avoid the transfer of microorganism contamination from one person to another. Which one of the following methods prevents cross infection from staff to patients?

  A Disinfection

  B Handwashing

  C Sterilisation

  D Zoning

9 Various methods are used in the dental workplace to prevent cross-infection incidents. Which one of the following options is the term used to describe the method of preventing contamination of equipment items that cannot be sterilised in the usual way?

A Barrier method

B Surface cleaning

C Use of disposables

D Zoning

10 The basic principle of the system of 'standard (universal) precautions' used in all health-care work environments is to assume which one of the following?

A All dental personnel will be free from disease

B All patients will have received a full range of childhood vaccinations

C Any patient may be infected with a pathogen at any time

D Any patient may have a natural immunity to some diseases

11 Which one of the following options is the term used when items have undergone a process to remove physical contamination so that they can be rendered safe for reuse?

A Cleaned

B Decontaminated

C Disinfected

D Sterilised

12 Which one of the following items of personal protective equipment is most important in preventing cross infection by aerosol spray?

A Mask

B Plastic apron

C Safety glasses

D Visor

13 There are various routes of transmission of microorganisms that may result in a cross-infection incident. Which one of the following options is the most likely route of transmission from a patient when a member of staff has an uncovered wound on their finger?

A Aerosol spray

B Airborne droplets

C Direct entry

D Inoculation

14 Hand hygiene is important in minimising the risk of cross infection in the dental workplace. Which level of hand hygiene aims to significantly reduce the numbers of normally resident microorganisms on the hands?

A Clinical

B Hygienic

C Social

D Surgical

15 There are various levels of cleanliness referred to in the clinical setting. Which one of the following options is the term used when all pathogenic microorganisms and spores have been destroyed by the cleaning method involved?

A Decontaminated

B Disinfected

C Socially clean

D Sterilised

16 Various methods are used in the dental workplace to prevent cross-infection incidents. Which one of the following options is the term used when dirty instruments are physically separated from clean ones during a dental procedure?

A Barrier method

B Surface cleaning

C Use of disposables

D Zoning

17 Which one of the following options identifies the reason for the use of sealed pouches to store instruments in the clinical area of the dental workplace?

A Allows easy identification of items

B Avoids aerosol contamination

C Keeps items dry

D Keeps items tidy

18 Which one of the following options is a suitable disinfectant for the routine cleaning of work surfaces in the clinical area between patients and for use as an impression disinfectant too?

A Aldehyde

B Chlorhexidine gluconate

C Isopropyl alcohol

D Sodium hypochlorite

19 Various items of equipment are used in the dental workplace to assist in infection control processes. Which one of the following items is used to sterilise instruments and render them safe for reuse?

A Autoclave

B Distiller

C Ultrasonic bath

D Washer–disinfector

20 Which one of the following statements regarding clinical handwashing technique is false?

A Antibacterial soap should be used

B Illustrated directions should be present at each handwashing sink

C Rinsing should occur towards the fingers

D Taps should not be hand operated

21 Which one of the following options summarises the need for standard precautions to be followed at all times in the dental workplace?

A Avoids identifying infectious patients

B Healthy carrier cannot be identified

C Helps isolate infectious patients

D Prevents any staff exposure to infectious patients

22 Indirect cross infection occurs when microorganisms are transferred from a contaminated item to another person. Which one of the following techniques will prevent the occurrence of indirect cross-infection incidents?

A Decontamination of items

B High-speed aspiration

C Use of disposables

D Zoning of the clinical area

23 Many viruses are transmitted from person to person by direct contact with infected blood. Which one of the following options is the correct chemical for use when cleaning away a blood spillage?

A Aldehyde

B Chlorhexidine gluconate

C Detergent

D Sodium hypochlorite

24 Which one of the following statements regarding the reprocessing of instruments is false?

A All instruments should be sterilised before reuse

B Detergent solution should be used when manually scrubbing instruments

C Endodontic files should be discarded after use

D Metal brushes should be used to remove persistent debris

25 Which one of the following options is the correct sequence of events to be followed during the decontamination of instruments before sterilisation is carried out?

A Debride, inspect, rinse and scrub

B Debride, scrub, rinse and inspect

C Scrub, inspect, rinse and debride

D Scrub, rinse, debride and inspect

Answers

1 *Correct answer C*: Social handwashing involves the use of general-purpose soap (rather than a special antibacterial hand cleanser) that is worked into a lather to physically clean the hands. This action will remove any general microorganisms from the hand surfaces, such as those acquired by using door handles in public places, taps and toilet flush handles and so on.

2 *Correct answer C*: Aerosol spray and particle spatter are everyday occurrences during the delivery of dental treatment and are always likely to occur in this environment. Direct contact with some body fluids (such as saliva or respiratory tract discharge) may occur outside of the immediate clinical area simply by contact with the public, as happens anywhere. However, inoculation injuries should be a rare occurrence if the infection control policy is followed correctly by all dental personnel.

3 *Correct answer A*: There are many diseases that can be transmitted without every sufferer becoming ill immediately (if at all), and the infected person is then often unaware that they have been exposed to pathogens. However, they can still pass the disease onto a third person by any of the usual routes of transmission, and that person will also then become infected. This intermediary who shows no signs of disease nor suffers any symptoms is called a carrier, and the likelihood of a healthy carrier unknowingly being treated at some point in a dental workplace forms the basis of the principles of 'standard precautions' – to treat every patient as a possible source of infection.

4 *Correct answer B*: This is the standard definition of disinfection, a cleaning process that usually involves the use of chemicals but that only kills some microorganisms, not all of them. Some viruses and the inactive state of bacteria (called spores) are unaffected by disinfection techniques and can be assumed to be present and infective unless more thorough cleaning methods are employed, such as sterilisation.

5 *Correct answer B*: Modern dental procedures often involve the use of high-speed hand pieces and ultrasonic instruments that create aerosols and throw particulate matter into the surrounding environment. As the spray produced falls down from the air, all exposed work surfaces can be assumed to become contaminated by any debris and pathogens within it, and they must be wiped over with a suitable surface disinfectant between patients to prevent cross infection.

6 *Correct answer B*: Indirect cross infection occurs when contamination from one patient is transferred to an instrument that is then used on a second patient without the contaminant being removed first. Extraction forceps are reusable items, but they must undergo sterilisation to be rendered safe for reuse on other patients. The process of disinfection alone will only remove bacteria, fungi and some viruses, and the forceps may therefore still harbour pathogens that are likely to infect the next patient.

7 *Correct answer C*: Disposable items are also referred to as single-use items – they are used on one patient and then safely disposed of, rather than undergoing a sterilisation process and used again on another patient. By disposing of an item after it has been used on just one patient, any contamination or pathogens it may harbour will never have the opportunity of infecting another patient because the item will never come into contact with another patient. The use of disposables is therefore the most effective method of preventing cross infection between patients.

8 *Correct answer B*: Handwashing is the main method of minimising the risk of cross infection from one person to another, as our hands come into contact with a multitude of potentially infected surfaces and items on a day-to-day basis, as well as being used for such personal events as nose blowing, self-cleaning after going to the toilet and so on. Of the options listed, handwashing is the only one that involves the removal of potential contamination from a staff member, while the other three options are all concerned with the removal of contamination from a patient after having undergone dental treatment.

9 *Correct answer A*: This technique involves covering large equipment items, or their control switches, with a layer of impervious membrane such as cling film. This prevents any direct contact of the equipment by dirty hands or by aerosol contamination during a dental procedure. Once the procedure has been completed, the barrier film is removed and safely disposed of, and a new layer can be placed before treatment begins on the next patient. Items protected in this way include computer keyboards, dental chair control switches, dental light handles and switches and the like.

10 *Correct answer C*: Therefore, every patient is always assumed to be potentially infected with a pathogen while attending for dental treatment and treated under standard precautions as if they could infect others at any time. Dental personnel will only be free from those diseases for which they have immunity, and all patients cannot be assumed to have received a full range of childhood vaccinations. A patient may have natural immunity to some diseases, but that will not protect dental personnel from infection by other pathogens.

11 *Correct answer B*: The items have been contaminated by body tissue and fluids from the patient during the course of their dental treatment. They are decontaminated by undergoing manual scrubbing or debridement in an ultrasonic bath or a washer–disinfector, so that the body tissue and fluids are removed from their surfaces. They can then undergo sterilisation to ensure that any pathogen contamination is killed before the items are safely reused on another patient.

12 *Correct answer A*: A face mask fits snugly over the nose and mouth when worn correctly and will prevent the inhalation of any aerosol spray. A visor protects the face from direct spatter created during dental procedures, but aerosol spray can still be inhaled around its open sides and beneath its open base, and it does not therefore adequately protect the staff member from this source of cross infection. Aerosol spray contamination is a cross-infection risk if inhaled, so the other options are not relevant.

13 *Correct answer C*: Normally, the intact skin surface is the first line of the body's natural defence mechanisms against entry by pathogens to cause an infection. An uncovered wound provides a site of direct entry to pathogens through the breach in the skin and directly into the deeper tissue layers. If the wound was covered with a waterproof dressing, this would act as a protective barrier while the skin healed beneath and would also act to prevent the entry of pathogens. Aerosol spray and airborne droplets usually gain entry by inhalation, while an inoculation route involves the piercing of intact skin by an infected sharp implement.

14 *Correct answer D*: Surgical handwashing involves the thorough and systematic cleaning of every area of the hands and forearms using a surgical-grade washing solution to significantly reduce the numbers of microorganisms that are normally resident on the skin in these areas. So this is over and above the removal of any acquired microorganisms that the person may also have become contaminated with in their normal activities. This level of hand hygiene is necessary when a person is involved in any invasive surgical procedures.

15 *Correct answer D*: This is the standard definition of the process of sterilisation, where not just the pathogens but their inactive spores are destroyed so that items cleaned in this way are termed as aseptic – devoid of all living microorganisms.

16 *Correct answer D*: This technique involves the designation of clearly marked sections of workspace within the clinical area – clean and dirty – that are strictly adhered to by all dental personnel working in that area. Only clean items are placed in the clean section, and only dirty items are placed in the dirty section, and the two areas are physically separated from each other in the layout of the clinical area so that there is no confusion. Often, this separation is achieved by having separate worktops in the two areas or by a sink or other such appliance placed between the two sections. The two areas will also be clearly labelled to avoid any mishaps.

17 *Correct answer B*: Even with sterilised items being placed in cupboards and drawers within the clinical area when not in use, there is always the potential for them to become contaminated by aerosol spray while dental procedures are being carried out in the near vicinity. The spray will always be created when hand pieces and ultrasonic scalers are used and may take some time to fall and land onto any available surfaces in the surgery – it will not be apparent because the spray is invisible. Sealing items in pouches provides a physical barrier to this potential source of contamination and guarantees their sterilised status when they are eventually opened and reused.

18 *Correct answer A*: Aldehyde is a powerful disinfectant against bacteria, fungi and some viruses and is used as pre-impregnated wipes for effective surface cleaning in the clinical area between patients. It can also be used in solution as an immersion bath for the disinfection of impressions. Sodium hypochlorite is a more powerful disinfectant still, but its choking smell and bleaching abilities make it unlikely to be used routinely throughout a working session. It tends to be reserved for deep cleaning and specialist incidents such as blood spillages when no other disinfectant is suitable. The other two options are not suitable disinfectants for either purpose stated.

19 *Correct answer A*: Autoclaves are pressure vessels that heat their contents to a set temperature under pressure and hold them in this state for a set time to ensure that all pathogens are killed. Some work under vacuum, while others draw the steam created during the process over the contents to ensure sterility. Ultrasonic baths act to decontaminate items and washer–disinfectors do as their name states. Distillers are used to convert tap water into distilled water that can then be used to operate these items of cleaning equipment.

20 *Correct answer C*: The fingers are the parts of the hand that will come into contact with patients and items or instruments and therefore need to be as clean as possible. By rinsing after clinical handwashing with the water flowing away from the fingers (rather than as stated in the question), all of the used soap solution and any contamination it contains will be guaranteed to be removed from the fingers so that they are clinically clean. All three of the other statements are true.

21 *Correct answer B*: A healthy carrier of a pathogenic disease will show no signs nor feel any symptoms of illness and will therefore be assumed to be non-infectious to others. However, they are infectious and can pass on the disease through the relevant transmission route to any person they come into contact with – this is how diseases can spread uncontrollably. The main principle of standard precautions is to assume that every person can be an unidentified healthy carrier of any disease and to treat every person as if they are just that. So full infection control procedures are used across the board when treating any patient, whether they show signs of illness or not, and the risk of transmission is reduced massively.

22 *Correct answer C*: If contaminated items are disposed of after a single use on one patient only, there is no risk of transmission to another person by reuse. None of the other options will prevent indirect cross-infection incidents.

23 *Correct answer D*: Sodium hypochlorite (bleach) at a 1% concentration is the only recommended solution to be used to clean away a blood spillage effectively. It is more effective against viruses (including HIV and hepatitis B) than aldehyde solution, and the other two options are not viricidal and must not be used for blood spillages.

24 *Correct answer D*: Microscopically, the use of metal brushes to remove persistent debris can cause scratching of the metal surface of instruments, which then makes them more likely to harbour pathogens when used again and therefore more likely to cause cross infection. All three of the other options are true.

25 *Correct answer A*: Debridement is performed by placing the items into either an ultrasonic bath or a washer–disinfector for the correct time period and using the correct chemicals. This renders the items safe to be handled while wearing clean PPE, so that they can be visually inspected for residual contamination, rinsed and then manually scrubbed to remove this contamination before being autoclaved.

OUTCOME 2

Understand the Significance of Microorganisms

Questions

1 Which one of the following types of infectious agent is present as protein capsules living within other body cells?
   A Bacteria
   B Fungi
   C Prions
   D Viruses

2 Which one of the following options is not one of the body's natural lines of defence against a disease caused by a bacterial infection?
   A Antibiotics
   B Immune response
   C Inflammatory response
   D Intact skin layer

3 Many bacteria are named according to the shape of their cells. Which one of the following options is a rod-shaped microorganism that is associated with established carious cavities in teeth?
   A Actinomyces
   B Lactobacilli
   C *Staphylococcus aureus*
   D *Streptococcus mutans*

4 Potentially infectious diseases are usually caused by a type of microorganism. Which one of the following is not a type of pathogenic microorganism?
   A Bacteria
   B Fungi
   C Prions
   D Viruses

Questions and Answers for Diploma in Dental Nursing, Level 3, First Edition. Carole Hollins.
© 2016 John Wiley & Sons, Ltd. Published 2016 by John Wiley & Sons, Ltd.

5 Infection occurs when pathogenic microorganisms gain entry to the body tissues. Which route of transmission is most likely to be involved when a dental nurse works with a colleague who has a common cold and is sneezing regularly?

A Aerosol transmission

B Airborne droplets

C Direct contact

D Inoculation injury

6 Which one of the following options is a fatal disease that affects the nerve tissues of the body?

A Acquired immune deficiency syndrome

B Creutzfeldt–Jakob disease

C Hepatitis C

D Swine influenza

7 Which one of the following statements best describes the difference between a pathogen and a non-pathogen?

A Non-pathogens are also known as prions

B Non-pathogens can cause non-fatal diseases

C Pathogens always cause fatal diseases

D Pathogens have the potential to cause disease, while non-pathogens do not

8 Which one of the following types of infectious agent is found as single-cell organisms that can exist in unfavourable environments as spores?

A Bacteria

B Fungi

C Prions

D Viruses

9 *Candida albicans* is a fungal microorganism that is found in several oral disease conditions. Which one of the following diseases is not associated with this fungal infection?

A Angular cheilitis

B Cold sore

C Denture stomatitis

D Oral thrush

10 There are various routes of transmission of microorganisms that enable them to cause disease in the body. Which one of the following options is the route that is the most likely to result in an infection?

A Aerosol spray

B Airborne droplets

C Direct contact

D Inoculation injury

11 When the skin or mucous membranes are breached by a pathogen, the body reacts by initiating an inflammatory response. Which one of the following is usually the last of the five signs of this response?

A Loss of function

B Pain

C Redness

D Swelling

12 Which one of the following options is the fatal disease caused by a viral infection that destroys the body's immune system and may cause several lesions not seen in other diseases?

A Acquired immune deficiency syndrome

B Hepatitis B

C Meningitis

D Poliomyelitis

13 Which group of drugs is available for use against an infection caused by a bacterial microorganism?

A Analgesics

B Antibiotics

C Antihistamines

D Anti-inflammatories

14 Many bacteria are named according to the shape of their cells. Which one of the following microorganisms is spiral shaped and is associated with an ulcerative periodontal infection?

A Actinomyces

B *Staphylococcus aureus*

C *Streptococcus mutans*

D *Treponema vincenti*

15 Infection occurs when pathogenic microorganisms gain entry to the body tissues. Which one of the following options is a potential route of transmission of infection that is especially likely in the dental workplace?

A Aerosol spray

B Airborne droplets

C Direct contact

D Direct entry

16 Which one of the following statements regarding the disease hepatitis B is false?

A It can be prevented by vaccination

B It is caused by a virus

C It is transmitted mainly in saliva

D It often results in primary liver cancer

17 Which one of the following types of infectious agent is found as microscopic plant-like organisms that reproduce by budding or by producing spores?

   A Bacteria

   B Fungi

   C Prions

   D Viruses

18 Many bacteria are named according to the shape of their cells. Which one of the following options is a round-shaped microorganism that is associated with dental caries?

   A Actinomyces

   B Lactobacilli

   C *Staphylococcus aureus*

   D *Streptococcus mutans*

19 A Patient may attend with a 'cold sore' lesion on their lip. Which one of the following statements about a cold sore lesion is true?

   A It is associated with the trigeminal nerve

   B It is caused by herpes varicella virus

   C It is not infectious

   D It is often a premalignant lesion

20 Which one of the following diseases cannot be prevented by vaccination?

   A Chickenpox

   B Hepatitis C

   C Tetanus

   D Tuberculosis

Answers

1 *Correct answer D*: These are ultramicroscopic organisms living within tissue cells and cause diseases such as hepatitis B. Bacteria exist as microscopic single-cell organisms, fungi exist as microscopic plant-like organisms, and prions are a type of specialised protein rather than a microorganism.

2 *Correct answer A*: Antibiotics are drugs that are taken to kill bacteria, but they are not naturally present in the body as a line of defence against diseases – they must be ingested. The first line of the body's natural defence is the physical barrier provided by the skin and mucous membranes. If these are breached, a localised inflammatory response is instigated, and if this fails to destroy the invading pathogens, then the body releases its immune response to fight them.

3 *Correct answer B*: Bacilli are classically rod shaped (like grains of rice), and lactobacilli are found deep in established carious cavities. Actinomyces are also bacilli, but are not associated with caries. Streptococci are circular in shape as a chain, while staphylococci occur as clusters of circular microorganisms.

4 *Correct answer C*: These are a type of specialised protein rather than a microorganism and cause infectious conditions such Creutzfeldt-Jakob disease (CJD). All three other options are examples of microorganisms.

5 *Correct answer B*: The infective microorganisms will be expelled from the colleague's nose during sneezing as airborne droplets, contaminating the surrounding environment and allowing their inhalation by others so that the disease is spread. Inhalation is the main entry route of the virus responsible for the common cold.

6 *Correct answer B*: This disease and its variants were identified in humans as being caused by infection with prion proteins and are similar to 'mad cow' disease found in cattle (bovine spongiform encephalopathy – BSE). It affects potentially any nerve tissue in the body, including the pulp tissue of the teeth, and has no cure. Its existence is the reason why endodontic instruments are now classed as single use and must not be reprocessed for use on other patients.

7 *Correct answer D*: This is the distinction between the two groups. Prions are specialised proteins that are capable of acting as pathogens and causing disease (such as CJD). Diseases are not always fatal – dental caries and periodontitis are diseases, but patients do not die of tooth decay nor gum disease.

8 *Correct answer A*: Bacteria are named according to the shape of their single cells (i.e., cocci, bacilli, spirochaete and so on) and live in colonies as clusters or chains, for example. When in their vegetative (non-active) state, they exist as spores and are able to withstand harsh environments such as temperature extremes or severe drought, in a similar way to plant seeds.

9 *Correct answer B*: Cold sores are caused by the herpes simplex virus and appear as a highly infectious, crusting lesion on the lip following the primary herpes infection, which may have occurred years previously. All three other options are associated with the *Candida albicans* fungus.

10 *Correct answer D*: The body has three lines of natural defence against infection – the physical barrier provided by the skin or membranes and their secretions, the inflammatory response and the immune response. An inoculation injury, by definition, has already bypassed the first line of defence so that pathogens have been placed deep within the body tissues. Only the remaining two responses can prevent infection from occurring in this case, whereas pathogens involved in the other three options must still breach the physical barrier before gaining entry to the deeper tissues.

11 *Correct answer A*: The increased blood flow to the area that occurs in the initial response of the body to the presence of the pathogen as a 'foreign invader' is responsible for the heat, redness and swelling that occur with inflammation. The swelling of the tissues caused by the increased blood flow presses on the surrounding nerves and causes the pain associated with inflammation. This pain then prevents the affected part of the body from being used as normal, because it is painful to do so – it undergoes a loss of function.

12 *Correct answer A*: Sufferers of acquired immune deficiency syndrome (AIDS) can often be infected for years before showing any signs of illness. The human immunodeficiency virus (HIV) involved gradually attacks and destroys their immune system so that they succumb to either commonplace infections, which would normally be survivable, or they suffer from unusual infections, which are rare and not normally seen in their population group. Quite often, AIDS is suspected in these cases when the sufferer develops unusual lesions that have become associated with the disease – one such being the oral lesion of Kaposi's sarcoma.

13 *Correct answer B*: Many different types of antibiotics are available for use against the vast array of bacteria that cause disease, although their overuse for mild diseases has led to strains of 'superbugs' developing (such as MRSA in hospitals), which are able to survive a course of treatment with conventional doses of antibiotics. Analgesics are used as painkillers, antihistamines are taken to reduce the body's over-response to some allergens (such as with hay fever and other allergies), and anti-inflammatories are taken to reduce inflammation.

14 *Correct answer D*: *Treponema vincenti* is the spirochaete (spiral shaped) bacterium associated with acute necrotising ulcerative gingivitis (ANUG). Actinomyces are rod-shaped bacilli, and the other two options are examples of round cocci bacteria.

15 *Correct answer A*: The other three options are routes of transmission that may occur anywhere, but aerosol spray is produced in abundance in the dental workplace while using high-speed turbines and ultrasonic instruments during dental procedures and is not commonplace outside of this environment. In the absence of the use of personal protective equipment and a robust infection control policy, infection by this route is quite possible for the dental staff.

16 *Correct answer C*: Hepatitis B is transmitted mainly in blood rather than saliva. All three of the other options are true.

17 *Correct answer B*: Fungi exist and appear microscopically as plant-like organisms similar to mushrooms and toadstools, with their fruiting bodies producing spores as a form of reproduction as well as by growing bud-like extensions of their main body that break off and produce a new fungal colony.

18 *Correct answer D*: Although not the only bacterium associated with dental caries, it is certainly the most prolific and the most likely to be identified in early carious lesions. Lactobacilli tend to colonise established carious lesions, and neither actinomyces nor staphylococci are associated with dental caries.

19 *Correct answer A*: These lesions are due to an initial infection with the herpes simplex virus that then lies dormant in the trigeminal nerve (fifth cranial nerve) and presents as a crusty lesion on the lip. This lesion is highly infectious, especially to the dental staff when an afflicted patient is receiving dental treatment, but it is not associated with premalignancy.

20 *Correct answer B*: There is currently no vaccination available to prevent hepatitis C infection, which causes chronic liver disease in the majority of its sufferers, often many years after their initial exposure. It is a blood-borne virus and is therefore a potential threat to the dental staff in the absence of a robust infection control policy and non-compliance with standard precautions in the clinical setting. Liver transplant usually offers the only hope of survival for many sufferers.

OUTCOME 3

Understand the Management of Infectious Conditions Affecting Dental Patients

Questions

1 Which of the following infectious conditions of a patient is most likely to infect a member of the dental team during normal chairside work?
   A Cold sore lesion
   B Dental caries
   C Hepatitis B
   D Mumps

2 Cross infection may occur from patient to staff and vice versa. Which one of the following infection control procedures is most likely to reduce cross infection from staff to patients?
   A Barrier membrane
   B Handwashing
   C Use of a face mask
   D Wearing gloves

3 The immune response is a normal occurrence when the body tissues have been invaded by microorganisms. Which one of the following are developed during this response to neutralise the poisons from the microorganisms?
   A Antibodies
   B Antigens
   C Antitoxins
   D Immunoglobulins

4 Which one of the following diseases presents as a swelling of either one or both parotid salivary glands, usually in children and young adults?
   A Measles
   B Mumps
   C Rubella
   D Tuberculosis

Questions and Answers for Diploma in Dental Nursing, Level 3, First Edition. Carole Hollins.
© 2016 John Wiley & Sons, Ltd. Published 2016 by John Wiley & Sons, Ltd.

5 Which of the following diseases must all clinical dental personnel be vaccinated against before working at the chairside?

A Acquired immune deficiency syndrome (AIDS)

B Creutzfeldt–Jakob disease

C Hepatitis B

D Hepatitis C

6 Which one of the following statements regarding the infectious disease hepatitis B is false?

A It can be killed by hypochlorite disinfectants

B It can survive immersion in boiling water

C It is less infective than human immunodeficiency virus (HIV)

D It is unaffected by chlorhexidine disinfectants

7 Which one of the following statements regarding immunisation is true?

A All vaccines result in lifelong immunity

B Hepatitis C is prevented by immunisation

C Living microorganisms may be used to provide immunity

D Vaccination results in natural immunity against a disease

8 Which one of the following infectious diseases affecting the head and neck region is usually caused by Epstein–Barr virus?

A Glandular fever

B Hand, foot and mouth disease

C Mumps

D Stomatitis

9 When a person is exposed to an infectious disease for a second time, their immune system will recognise the microorganisms and act to fight the invasion. Which one of the following will be released against the invaders during the immune response mechanism?

A Antibodies

B Antigens

C Antitoxins

D Toxins

10 Which one of the following options is the most likely infection control method to prevent indirect cross infection from one patient to another?

A Handwashing

B Sterilisation

C Use of full PPE

D Use of single-use disposables

11 Which one of the following infections presents as generalised stomatitis with many shallow painful ulcers present and which takes up to 14 days to resolve?

A Glandular fever

B Oral thrush

C Primary herpes simplex

D Shingles

12 Clinical/hygienic handwashing should be carried out by the dental team several times a day while treating patients. Which of the following is the minimum length of time that the actual handwashing process with antibacterial soap should take?

A 10 s

B 20 s

C 30 s

D 60 s

13 Which one of the following infectious conditions does not present with any oral manifestations?

A Hepatitis B

B Herpes simplex

C Measles

D Tuberculosis

14 Which one of the following statements regarding immunisation and the immune system is false?

A Erythrocytes are released during the immune response

B Immunisation results in antibodies against fatal diseases

C Immunoglobulins are present in saliva

D Some people have natural immunity to diseases

15 Which one of the following options is the most likely infection control method to prevent direct cross infection from one patient to another?

A Handwashing

B Sterilisation

C Wearing gloves

D Zoning

16 Which one of the following options is a known risk factor for a person to be a carrier of Creutzfeldt–Jakob disease or variant Creutzfeldt–Jakob disease?

A Drug addiction

B Family history

C History of institutionalisation

D Sexual promiscuity

17 Immunity from certain diseases is important in protecting dental personnel from contracting potentially life-threatening conditions from their patients. What is the term used to describe the type of protection that is inherited from one's mother?

A Acquired immunity

B Live vaccine

C Natural immunity

D Passive immunity

18 Healthy members of the dental team are unlikely to contract an infection in the workplace if they take suitable precautions and their natural defence mechanisms are intact. Which of the following events will involve leucocytes fighting the pathogenic microorganism once a dental nurse has been exposed to them?

A Inflammatory response mechanism

B Immune response mechanism

C Intact skin and mucous membranes

D Personal protective equipment

19 Which one of the following options is a viral disease that is usually transmitted by saliva from one person to another?

A Acquired immune deficiency syndrome

B Chickenpox

C Hepatitis B

D Mumps

20 Which one of the following chemicals should be used to clean away a blood spillage in the dental workplace?

A Aldehyde

B Chlorhexidine gluconate

C Isopropyl alcohol

D Sodium hypochlorite

21 Which one of the following actions should be carried out to ensure that dental staff and patients are not exposed to blood-borne viral diseases in the dental workplace?

A Follow standard precautions

B Refer carriers to hospital for dental treatment

C Treat infectious patients at the session end

D Use a vacuum autoclave

Answers

1 *Correct answer A*: This common infectious condition is caused by a virus and produces highly infectious lip lesions that may infect clinical dental staff during the provision of dental treatment. Dental staff will be vaccinated against hepatitis B and mumps, and dental caries is not infectious.

2 *Correct answer B*: Handwashing by staff will reduce the normally present microorganisms they have on their own skin, as well as remove any microorganisms present that they have acquired during their normal daily duties. These contaminants cannot then be passed on to patients. Personal protective equipment is worn to prevent staff from becoming infected by patients, and barrier membranes are used to prevent the contamination of equipment items that cannot undergo sterilisation, such as overhead lights and bracket table control panels.

3 *Correct answer C*: The poisons produced by the microorganisms are called toxins, and once they have been identified and recognised by the body's immune system, it releases the necessary antitoxins to neutralise them. This limits the damage that the invading microorganisms cause to the body tissues and allows the immune system to successfully defeat the pathogens. Antibodies (of which immunoglobulins are an example) are produced by the immune system to fight the actual pathogen, and antigens are the actual agents that initiate the immune response and stimulate the production of antibodies – so they may be microorganisms (as in this context), pollen grains, chemicals and so on.

4 *Correct answer B*: Mumps is an infection of the parotid salivary gland only (one or both) due to the paramyxovirus; it does not affect the other salivary glands. It usually occurs in childhood in those who have not been vaccinated against it during routine childhood inoculation programmes but is more serious if it occurs in adults as male infertility can result. Rubella is also known as German measles.

5 *Correct answer C*: All clinical dental personnel must be vaccinated against this highly infective blood-borne viral disease, as they are at risk of exposure during normal dental procedures. There are no vaccines available against the other three options.

6 *Correct answer C*: Hepatitis B is far more infective than HIV, and it is estimated that one person in every 1000 is a carrier of the virus – so dental staff are very likely to come into contact with infected individuals many times during their careers. All three of the other options are true.

7 *Correct answer C*: Living microorganisms are often required to be used in vaccines to allow the body to develop a suitable immune response against the disease they cause, but they have to be altered in some way beforehand so that the recipient does not go on to develop the full-blown disease they cause and risk death. All three of the other options are false.

8 *Correct answer A*: Correctly known as infectious mononucleosis, glandular fever is a viral infection presenting as a debilitating fever and sore throat in adolescents, often with swollen glands in the neck and armpits. Hand, foot and mouth disease is due to infection with coxsackievirus, and mumps is due to infection with paramyxovirus. Stomatitis is a general term for inflammation of the soft tissues of the oral cavity.

9 *Correct answer A*: Antibodies are the proteins produced by the immune system in direct response to the presence of a specific antigen – a certain microorganism, another foreign body such as pollen grains, a chemical and so on. They act to fight the antigen and destroy it, so that the disease or effect they produce is destroyed. Some infectious microorganisms produce toxins during their attack on the body, and the immune response develops antitoxins to neutralise them.

10 *Correct answer D*: Indirect cross infection occurs when a patient contaminates an item or instrument that is then used on another patient. If items are classed as single use and disposed of once they have been used on one patient only, there can be no transfer of infection to another patient. While sterilisation should render all items safe if they are autoclaved, there is always the possibility that they have not been correctly decontaminated first, so a theoretical risk exists that indirect cross infection can occur under these circumstances. Handwashing and the use of PPE are concerned with the transfer of contamination from or to staff members, respectively.

11 *Correct answer C*: Primary herpes simplex infection can occur at any age and can be mild enough to go unnoticed but usually presents in the way described. The virus then lies dormant in the trigeminal nerve and may represent as cold sores on the lips for the rest of life. Glandular fever and shingles do not affect the oral cavity, and the fungal infection of oral thrush presents as a white coating of the soft tissues that can be removed to reveal a red, bleeding base.

12 *Correct answer C*: This is the minimum recommended time required to wash all areas of the hands in the correct manner, as displayed on the handwashing posters that must be present at each designated sink. Sixty seconds is more than sufficient time to carry out the procedure effectively.

13 *Correct answer A*: This disease affects the liver. Herpes simplex presents as multiple areas of oral ulceration, measles sufferers display lesions on the insides of the cheeks (Koplik's spots), and tuberculosis presents as a gradually increasing deep and painful ulcer, commonly located at the back of the surface (dorsum) of the tongue.

14 *Correct answer A*: Erythrocytes are red blood cells and are involved in the transport of oxygen from the lungs to the rest of the body in the circulatory system. It is the white blood cells (leucocytes) that are involved in the immune system and the defence of the body from attack by pathogens. All of the other three options are true.

15 *Correct answer B*: The process of sterilisation destroys all pathogens and their spores that have contaminated items and instruments after their use on a patient and involves the use of high temperatures and pressure in an autoclave (some also work under vacuum). Once sterilised, the items and instruments can be safely used again on another patient. Handwashing prevents contamination of a patient by a staff member, wearing gloves protects a staff member from contamination by a patient, and zoning restricts the contamination of clean items by dirty items during a dental procedure.

16 *Correct answer B*: The disease is caused by prions rather than living microorganisms and is passed directly in non-family members by infected nerve tissue following surgical procedures (theoretically including endodontic treatment). CJD is not a blood-borne disease and is not contracted by simple contact with an infected individual.

17 *Correct answer D*: This type of immunity is directly inherited from the mother. Acquired immunity is that given to a person by an inoculation programme (such as with hepatitis B) or developed by the immune system of the individual following exposure to the disease (such as with chickenpox). Natural immunity is that present from birth simply by random inheritance, and live vaccine is a type of inoculation using a living pathogen that has been rendered harmless before its use.

18 *Correct answer A*: This is the localised action of the infected body tissues to transport leucocytes (white blood cells) directly to the area so that they can fight and destroy the pathogens. The immune response involves other specialised leucocytes that do not fight the pathogens directly but are stimulated to release antibodies and antitoxins against the microorganisms. The skin and mucous membranes create physical barriers to the initial entry of the pathogens, and PPE is an applied method of prevention of the microorganisms from gaining entry to the body tissues.

19 *Correct answer D*: Acquired immune deficiency syndrome and hepatitis B are blood-borne viruses (although they are found in other body fluids), and chickenpox is transmitted by gaining entry through the mucosa of the respiratory tract by inhalation, airborne droplets or aerosol spray.

20 *Correct answer D*: Sodium hypochlorite (bleach) is the only suitable chemical shown for use in cleaning away a blood spillage. Aldehyde is a good disinfectant but is not active against several viruses that are able to be killed by bleach. The other two options have limited activity against most viruses.

21 *Correct answer A*: By treating every patient as a potential source of fatal pathogens (i.e. by following standard precautions), all dental staff should be safe from the possibility of disease transmission in the work environment.

OUTCOME 4

Know the Various Methods of Decontamination

Questions

1 Various methods are used in the dental workplace to help prevent the microorganism contamination of equipment and instruments. Which one of the following processes is used to kill all microorganisms and spores to produce asepsis?
   A Decontamination
   B Disinfection
   C Social cleaning
   D Sterilisation

2 When preparing reusable dental instruments for sterilisation, the correct sequence of cleaning actions must be followed to prevent cross infection. Which of the following options shows the correct sequence?
   A Debride, inspect, rinse and scrub
   B Debride, scrub, rinse and inspect
   C Scrub, inspect, rinse and debride
   D Scrub, rinse, debride and inspect

3 Once reusable items have been sterilised, they are sealed in windowed pouches and date-stamped. Which one of the following options correctly describes the system to be used for date-stamping a pair of extraction forceps?
   A Use by 1 year from date
   B Use by 21 days from date
   C Use by date shown (1 year hence)
   D Use by date shown (21 days hence)

Questions and Answers for Diploma in Dental Nursing, Level 3, First Edition. Carole Hollins.
© 2016 John Wiley & Sons, Ltd. Published 2016 by John Wiley & Sons, Ltd.

4 An ultrasonic bath is a device used during the cleaning procedure of reusable items in the dental workplace. Which one of the following options is most likely to result in a persistent failure of the ultrasonic bath to debride the items?

A Overloaded chamber

B Short vibration time

C Use of tap water

D Weak detergent solution

5 With regard to the manual cleaning of reusable items, which one of the following statements is false?

A Cleaning method is easily validated

B Items must be scrubbed under solution surface

C Items will require autoclaving before reuse

D Tap water is unsuitable for rinsing

6 A washer–disinfector is used in some dental workplaces to debride and disinfect reusable items before sterilisation. Which one of the following options shows the correct sequence of stages in the machine's cycle?

A Disinfect, flush, rinse, wash and dry

B Flush, wash, rinse, disinfect and dry

C Rinse, disinfect, flush, wash and dry

D Wash, rinse, disinfect, flush and dry

7 What is the purpose of carrying out a Helix test with regard to the use of autoclaves in the dental workplace?

A Ensure adequate pressure is reached

B Ensure adequate temperature is reached

C Ensure correct cycle time occurs

D Ensure steam penetration occurs

8 What is the term used to describe the technique of separating clean and contaminated areas in the clinical environment to avoid cross infection?

A Aspirating

B Barrier protecting

C Decontaminating

D Zoning

9 Which one of the following agents specifically cannot be used to disinfect metallic surfaces in the clinical environment?

A Aldehyde solution

B Chlorhexidine gluconate

C Sodium hypochlorite solution

D Viricidal wipes

10 Which one of the following options is not an example of industrial or large-scale sterilisation techniques?

A 'S'-type autoclave sterilisation

B Ethylene gas exposure

C Gamma irradiation

D Ultraviolet irradiation

11 The use of a decontamination room that is separate from the clinical area is the ideal situation in the dental workplace for the reprocessing of items and instruments. Within this room, which one of the following options describes the correct direction of airflow to avoid cross-contamination?

A Autoclave to instrument wash sink

B Ultrasonic bath to autoclave

C Washer–disinfector to autoclave

D Washer–disinfector to packaging area

12 Various chemicals are used to clean the clinical environment and reduce the risk of cross infection. Which one of the following is a routine use of the chemical isopropyl alcohol?

A Disinfection of impressions

B Hand cleanser

C Wiping exposed X-ray film packets

D Clearing small blood spillages

13 Various types of autoclave are available for use in the sterilisation of items and instruments. Which one of the following options describes the difference in the working action of an 'N'-type autoclave from a 'B'-type autoclave?

A Contents may be dried during cycle

B Downward displacement of steam

C Heats to 134°C and holds for 3 min

D Use of a vacuum

14 Various chemicals are used to achieve adequate cleaning and help prevent cross infection in the dental workplace. Which one of the following chemicals has been linked to hypersensitivity reactions in some patients and staff?

A Aldehyde

B Chlorhexidine

C Isopropyl alcohol

D Sodium hypochlorite

15 What is the term used to describe the technique of protecting non-sterilisable items from cross infection by the use of impervious membranes?

A Barrier protection

B Debridement

C Use of PPE

D Zoning

16 During the cleaning of reusable items following a dental procedure, all solid
debris must be removed from their surfaces. Which one of the following
techniques will not remove solid debris from items?

A Autoclave

B Manual scrubbing

C Ultrasonic bath

D Washer–disinfector

17 While cleaning the clinical environment, various chemicals are used to inhibit
the growth of, or ideally kill, bacteria and fungi. What is the correct term for
this procedure?

A Cleaning

B Decontamination

C Disinfection

D Sterilisation

18 Various items used during the provision of dental treatment are considered
to be single use and therefore disposable. Which one of the following items
may be reused following suitable sterilisation?

A Aspirator

B Barbed broach

C Matrix band

D Polishing brush

19 Which one of the following options regarding the preparation of the clinical
area to control cross infection is true?

A A lidded box should be available for the placement of dirty instruments
after use

B Bagged items should remain in a drawer until required during the
procedure

C Previously used instruments may remain in the dirty sink until the end of
the session

D Work surfaces should be covered with a barrier membrane

20 Which one of the following chemical decontaminants is found in skin cleansing
products for use in the clinical area?

A Aldehyde

B Chlorhexidine

C Isopropyl alcohol

D Sodium hypochlorite

21 Various types of autoclave are available for use in the sterilisation of items and instruments. Which one of the following options describes the difference in the working action of a 'B'-type autoclave from an 'N'-type autoclave?
A Contents must be pre-packaged
B Downward displacement of steam
C Holds for 3 min at a 2.2 bar pressure
D Use of a vacuum

22 During the decontamination of the clinical area after a dental procedure, work surfaces are wiped down to remove potential contamination by microorganisms such as those causing diseases, for example, hepatitis. Which one of the following options describes the action of these cleaning agents?
A Bactericidal
B Bacteriostatic
C Decontaminant
D Viricidal

23 Which one of the following items may not be sterilised if it is taken through a downward displacement autoclave cycle?
A Aspirating tip
B Burnisher
C Diamond bur
D Luxator

24 Before a dental procedure is carried out, the clinical area must be correctly prepared to limit the likelihood of cross infection occurring. Which one of the following options describes the method used to avoid contamination of clean items by soiled items?
A Barrier protection
B Disinfection
C Use of PPE
D Zoning

25 Which one of the following options is an example of a direct cross-infection incident?
A Contact with a dirty sink tap
B Dirty inoculation injury
C Inhalation of aerosol in a clinical area
D Reuse of a decontaminated paste filler

Answers

1 *Correct answer D*: Sterilisation is the only cleaning method available that kills all microorganisms and spores. Disinfection is not effective against all viruses and does not kill spores. Decontamination removes debris from items, while social cleaning is the most basic level of cleaning that simply physically removes any socially acquired microorganisms.

2 *Correct answer A*: Debridement is performed by placing the items into either an ultrasonic bath or a washer–disinfector for the correct time period and using the correct chemicals. This renders the items safe to be handled while wearing clean PPE, so that they can be visually inspected for residual contamination, rinsed and then manually scrubbed to remove this contamination before being autoclaved.

3 *Correct answer C*: This allows the system to run in line with other 'use by' products, such as foods and dental materials, therefore making life simpler for all involved. If the 'use by 1 year from date' system is used, the end date needs to be thought about and worked out, whereas the 'use by date shown' is quite straightforward – when that date arrives (or preferably just before), all packaged items must be sterilised, repackaged and newly stamped. The 21-day timeline was removed when HTM 01-05 was updated in 2013.

4 *Correct answer A*: Overloading the chamber prevents the ultrasonic vibrations from being transmitted to all the items within the bath, so that any debris they hold is not dislodged. This will happen every time the chamber is overloaded. While a short vibration time, use of tap water and a weak detergent solution are not ideal, some debris removal will still be achieved by the ultrasonic effect of the bath even under these circumstances.

5 *Correct answer A*: Validation is the term used to describe a system of authenticating, or proving, that something has happened. In this context, electronic items used in the decontamination of instruments and items use printouts, log data and items such as TST strips to prove that they have worked effectively during use – autoclaves and washer–disinfectors in particular use these methods. However, with manual cleaning, there is no system of validation available – the items either look clean to the person scrubbing them, or they do not and are then scrubbed again, and these actions are not recorded.

6 *Correct answer B*: Debridement (removal) of solid debris by flushing and washing must occur before successful disinfection can take place; otherwise, any debris remaining when the items undergo the disinfection stage will potentially protect any remaining microorganisms beneath the debris from the disinfection process. The items will then still be contaminated when they are placed into the autoclave and will then be a real cross-infection risk to the next patient who undergoes treatment with them.

7 *Correct answer D*: This is a test that must be carried out every day that the 'B'-type (vacuum) autoclave is used to ensure that the steam produced during the cycle does penetrate to the inside of any packaging used to enclose items or instruments – if it does not, then they cannot be assumed to be sterilised. A dated validation record is produced for each test that must be kept in the logbook for the autoclave. An alternative to the Helix test is the Bowie–Dick test. The other three options are all tested by the use of TST strips (or suitable alternatives).

8 *Correct answer D*: This technique uses a system of spatial separation between the areas where clean and dirty items are placed on the work surface within the clinical area, clearly marked by signage so that there is no confusion. All items that have been used on the patient and are then no longer required are placed directly into the dirty area – this may be the lidded box used to transfer the items into the decontamination area, where one is in use. They must not be removed from this area and reused during the course of treatment. All clean items in use during the same procedure are placed in a completely separate area, such as on the bracket table ready for use.

9 *Correct answer C*: Sodium hypochlorite (bleach) is corrosive to metals and must not be used to disinfect any metallic surfaces within the surgery. Both aldehyde solution and pre-impregnated viricidal wipes are suitable for the purpose instead. Chlorhexidine gluconate has no detrimental effect on metallic surfaces, but it is not suitable for use as a surface disinfectant.

10 *Correct answer D*: Ultraviolet radiation has long since been discredited as a suitable method of disinfecting items and instruments, let alone sterilising them. UV boxes could often be found in premises such as beauty salons, where they were used to 'disinfect' items used for manicures, pedicures and eyebrow shaping between customers. All three of the other options are correct.

11 *Correct answer A*: The airflow must travel from the clean zone of the decontamination room, where the autoclave and packaging areas are positioned, to the dirty zone where the contaminated instruments and items are first placed. It is simply achieved by placing an extractor fan in the dirty zone so that air is pulled into that area rather than expelled from it. The aim is to ensure that any potential airborne contamination in the room (from the reprocessing of dirty instruments) never moves across to the clean zone where sterilised items are being handled. All three of the other options have the airflow travelling in the opposite direction.

12 *Correct answer C*: Saliva contamination is removed from the packet with isopropyl alcohol wipes before being safely handled while wearing clean gloves. Isopropyl alcohol is not suitable for use as a disinfectant in any of the other three options.

13 *Correct answer B*: The 'N'-type autoclave works by reaching the appropriate temperature and pressure for the correct amount of time while pulling the steam generated down and over the contents of the chamber to sterilise them – hence the term 'downward displacement'. 'B'-type autoclaves ensure sterility by creating a vacuum within the chamber during the cycle. Both types of autoclave have the same working parameters, and both are able to be set to dry their contents at the end of the cycle.

14 *Correct answer B*: Chlorhexidine gluconate has been successfully used as the active ingredient in oral health products designed to treat periodontal disease for many years. More recently, its use has expanded to include irrigation during endodontic treatment, as well as inclusion in antibacterial soap solutions for use in the clinical environment. This increase in use has coincided with increasing reports of hypersensitivity reactions to various products containing the disinfectant, and patients should be carefully questioned before they are advised to use any products containing chlorhexidine.

15 *Correct answer A*: An impervious membrane such as cling film and other soft plastics is used to cover areas of large equipment items that are likely to be touched (and therefore contaminated) during a dental procedure. Such areas are the control panels of bracket tables, the tubing of handpieces, scalers, aspirators and the overhead dental light, which often requires readjustment during a procedure. These items cannot be sterilised in an autoclave, and merely wiping them down with a disinfectant solution after use may not be sufficient to remove all contamination. Consequently, they are covered by a membrane that prevents any solid or fluid movement through it (impervious), and this is removed, disposed of and replaced after each use.

16 *Correct answer A*: The autoclave is used to sterilise the reusable items once they have been decontaminated by any one of the other three options first. It does not act to physically remove any solid debris from items; indeed, the steam cannot penetrate this debris if any is present, and the items will not be sterile after the autoclave cycle is completed. All three of the other options are suitable methods of debridement.

17 *Correct answer C*: Disinfection involves the use of certain chemicals that act to inhibit the growth of some microorganisms or ideally to kill them. They are active against bacteria, fungi and some (but not all) viruses, and they have no effect on bacterial spores.

18 *Correct answer A*: Although the vast majority of aspirator tips used nowadays are single-use disposable plastic types, there are still some reusable types available that are made of metal (for surgical use) or a hard and shaped plastic (for high-speed aspiration). As they are hollow items, they must be sterilised in a vacuum autoclave to ensure that the inner surface of their lumen is fully exposed to the sterilisation process – this cannot be guaranteed to happen in downward displacement autoclaves. All three of the other options are classed as single use and disposable.

19 *Correct answer A*: The lidded box is used to safely transfer the contaminated items from the clinical area to the decontamination area (which should be two separate areas) without risk of contaminating the route while doing so, especially by dripping fluids along the way. Previously used items are placed into this box as they are finished during the procedure, rather than into the dirty sink. Bagged items that will be required during the procedure should be placed on the work surface for ease of access – if they are left in the drawer, then there is a risk of contaminating the other contents while collecting them during the procedure, or PPE must be constantly removed and replaced while collecting the items. Work surfaces do not require coverage with a barrier membrane, they are wiped down after each procedure.

20 *Correct answer B*: Chlorhexidine gluconate is a powerful disinfectant when in direct contact with body tissues and is used in many oral health products as an active ingredient against the various bacteria associated with periodontal disease. More recently, it has been added to various antibacterial liquid soaps for use in the clinical environment.

21 *Correct answer D*: The 'B'-type autoclave sterilises items under vacuum during the cycle and is therefore suitable for the sterilisation of hollow items such as aspirator tips, saliva ejectors and various items of surgical and implant kits. As the steam is pulled out of the chamber during the creation of the vacuum, it is drawn over and through every item in the chamber, ensuring that all microorganisms and spores are killed. The contents can be pre-packaged, but they do not have to be, and both types of autoclave work at this pressure and holding time. 'N'-type autoclaves work by downward displacement of the steam.

22 *Correct answer D*: Hepatitis B is a disease caused by the blood-borne virus of the same name, and the chemicals required to kill it and other viruses are termed viricidal (virus killing). Bactericidal agents kill bacteria, while bacteriostatic solutions inhibit the growth of bacteria, rather than killing them. Decontaminants remove debris from contaminated sites and items.

23 *Correct answer A*: An aspirator tip is a hollow item that requires sterilisation in a vacuum autoclave. The downward displacement of steam in an 'N'-type autoclave may not fully penetrate the inside of the aspirator, and it will not therefore be sterilised. All three of the other options are solid items and are able to be sterilised by the downward displacement process.

24 *Correct answer D*: Zoning is the technique of having clearly marked 'clean' and 'dirty' zones within the clinical area, where items and instruments may be safely placed to ensure there is no crossover of the two. So dirty items are never placed in the clean zone, and vice versa. This avoids cross infection of the clean items by any potential contamination from the dirty items.

25 *Correct answer B*: A dirty inoculation injury involves the direct transfer of contamination from one person into the body tissues of a second person, usually as a sharps injury by an instrument or needle that has been used on a patient and mishandled by a member of staff. The contamination does not have to fight through the skin or mucous membrane of the injured party to cause infection as would normally occur, as it has been deposited directly into the underlying tissues during the injury. All three of the other options are examples of indirect cross-infection incidents.

OUTCOME 5

Understand Relevant Health and Safety Legislation, Policies and Guidelines

Questions

1 Various regulations and legislation apply to the safe running of the dental workplace. Which one of the following options is the concern of the COSHH regulations?

  A Accidents at work
  B Chemicals
  C Fire extinguishers
  D Pressure vessels

2 The infection control policy in each dental workplace is followed to minimise the risk of cross infection between any persons in the premises. Which one of the following entries should be present specifically to protect staff from being infected by a patient?

  A Do not reuse disposable items
  B Follow handwashing instructions
  C Sterilise instruments correctly
  D Wear PPE correctly

3 Which one of the following options summarises the need for standard precautions to be followed at all times in the dental workplace?

  A Avoids offending infectious patients
  B Healthy carrier cannot be identified
  C Helps isolate infectious patients
  D Prevents any staff exposure to infectious patients

Questions and Answers for Diploma in Dental Nursing, Level 3, First Edition. Carole Hollins.
© 2016 John Wiley & Sons, Ltd. Published 2016 by John Wiley & Sons, Ltd.

4 The carrying out of a risk assessment is a routine event in the dental workplace to ensure the health and safety of all persons on the premises. Which one of the following actions should be the first stage of those listed?
   A Control the risk
   B Evaluate the risk
   C Identify the risk
   D Identify those at risk

5 Which one of the following disinfectant chemicals should be used to remove blood spatter following a dental procedure?
   A Aldehyde
   B Chlorhexidine gluconate
   C Isopropyl alcohol
   D Sodium hypochlorite

6 Which one of the following actions is the first that should be taken following a contaminated sharps injury?
   A Bleed the wound
   B Check the patient history
   C Cover the wound
   D Wash the wound

7 Which of the following items of personal protective equipment will protect the airway from aerosol contamination?
   A Face mask
   B Nitrile gloves
   C Safety glasses
   D Visor

8 Which one of the following waste disposal options is used to categorise and segregate out-of-date luting cements in the dental workplace?
   A Infectious waste
   B Non-hazardous waste
   C Non-infectious waste
   D Offensive waste

9 The process used to remove contamination from reusable items is called decontamination and involves four stages. Which one of the following is the first stage of this process to be carried out?
   A Cleaning
   B Disinfection
   C Inspection
   D Sterilisation

10 A washer–disinfector may be used in some dental workplaces as part of the infection control process. Before drying the contained items, which one of the following options is the first stage of the decontamination process with this machine?
   A Flush
   B Rinse
   C Thermal disinfection
   D Wash

11 The lead foil found within X-ray film packets will be handled under which one of the following waste categories?
   A Infectious waste
   B Non-hazardous waste
   C Non-infectious waste
   D Trade waste

12 Various tests must be carried out on a regular basis to ensure the correct working of equipment used to control cross infection. Which one of the following items must undergo a protein residue test on a weekly basis?
   A Downward displacement autoclave
   B Ultrasonic bath
   C Vacuum autoclave
   D Washer–disinfector

13 While carrying out a risk assessment, the likelihood of the subject under investigation to cause harm to someone is considered. Which one of the following options is the term used to describe this part of the risk assessment process?
   A Controlling
   B Evaluation
   C Identification
   D Recording

14 Gloves must be worn by all dental personnel when working at the chairside. Which one of the following options is the type of glove least suitable to be worn for these clinical procedures?
   A Latex
   B Nitrile
   C Powdered
   D Vinyl

15 Which one of the following statements with regard to autoclaves is false?
   A Downward displacement types can undergo control tests using 'TST' strips (or similar)
   B Downward displacement types operate at 134°C

   C Vacuum types are able to sterilise items that have not been decontaminated first

   D Vacuum types can sterilise hollow items

16 Various regulations and legislation apply to the safe running of the dental workplace. Which one of the following options is concerned with the consequences following an explosion of the autoclave?

   A COSHH

   B HTM 01-05

   C IR(ME)R

   D RIDDOR

17 The Special Waste and Hazardous Waste Regulations determine how all wastes in the dental workplace should be segregated and disposed of safely. Into which one of the following categories of waste may a sound extracted tooth be placed before collection and disposal?

   A Infectious waste (sharps)

   B Non-hazardous waste

   C Non-infectious waste

   D Offensive waste

18 A washer–disinfector may be used in some dental workplaces as part of the infection control process. Before drying the contained items, which one of the following options is the final stage of the decontamination process with this machine?

   A Flush

   B Rinse

   C Thermal disinfection

   D Wash

19 When a contaminated sharps injury occurs involving a high-risk patient, a microbiologist should be consulted with regard to the need for antiviral treatment to begin. Which one of the following options states where this person's contact details must be held in the dental workplace?

   A At reception

   B COSHH file

   C Infection control policy

   D RIDDOR file

20 Which one of the following items of personal protective equipment is not necessary to be worn during the reprocessing of contaminated instruments?

   A Face mask

   B Glasses

C Nitrile gloves
D Plastic apron

21 The process used to remove contamination from reusable items is called decontamination and involves four stages. Which one of the following is the final stage of this process to be carried out?
A Cleaning
B Disinfection
C Inspection
D Sterilisation

22 The carrying out of a risk assessment is a routine event in the dental workplace to ensure the health and safety of all persons on the premises. Which one of the following actions should be the final stage of those listed?
A Control the risk
B Evaluate the risk
C Identify the risk
D Identify those at risk

23 Which one of the following is the acceptable length of time that sterilised items may be stored away from the clinical area without being bagged in accordance with HTM 01-05?
A 1 day
B 1 week
C 1 year
D 21 days

24 Devices such as autoclaves act most efficiently when they are maintained correctly. Which one of the following options describes a maintenance action that should be carried out on a weekly basis for all autoclaves?
A Automatic control test
B Check door seal
C Empty water reservoir
D Steam penetration test

25 Legionnaires' disease is a respiratory condition that is associated with contaminated water supplies. Which one of the following options states the legislation/regulations under which this disease is a notifiable occurrence in the dental workplace?
A COSHH
B Environmental Protection Act
C Hazardous Waste Regulations
D RIDDOR

Answers

1 *Correct answer B*: The full title of these regulations is the Control of Substances Hazardous to Health, and they are concerned with the safe use of chemicals within the dental workplace. They require a risk assessment to be carried out of every chemical used in the premises – from cleaning products through dental materials and drugs to items such as correction fluid used in office administration tasks. The written reports produced have to be kept in a file for access by all staff in the event of an accident involving a chemical, so that first aid and professional advice can be given as necessary. Accidents at work including those involving pressure vessels are the realm of RIDDOR, and the use of fire extinguishers is controlled under the Fire Precaution Regulations.

2 *Correct answer D*: The wearing of items of personal protective equipment is necessary to ensure that contamination from a patient does not gain entry into the body tissues of a member of staff – by inhalation, ingestion, inoculation or by direct entry through the mucous membranes or surface wounds of the skin. All three of the other options are methods of protecting patients from contamination.

3 *Correct answer B*: A healthy carrier of a pathogenic disease will show no signs nor feel any symptoms of illness and will therefore be assumed to be non-infectious to others. However, they are infectious and can pass on the disease through the relevant transmission route to any person they come into contact with – this is how diseases can spread uncontrollably. The main principle of standard precautions is to assume that every person can be an unidentified healthy carrier of any disease and to treat every person as if they are just that. So full infection control procedures are used across the board when treating any patient, whether they show signs of illness or not, and the risk of transmission is reduced massively.

4 *Correct answer C*: The assessment cannot be carried out until the particular risk has been identified, so this has to be the first stage. The second stage is to identify who may be at risk, the third stage is to evaluate what the risk actually is, and the fourth stage is to control the risk accordingly so that all persons are safe.

5 *Correct answer D*: Sodium hypochlorite (bleach) is the only disinfectant listed that is suitable for cleaning away blood spillages, as it is active against the vast majority of viruses. All of the other three options are not suitable alternatives to bleach for this purpose.

6 *Correct answer A*: The wound should be squeezed and bled immediately to remove any potential contamination at the injury site before it has a chance to get into the victim's bloodstream. The wound can then be washed, dried, and covered with a dressing, and then the patient history can be accessed to determine the level of risk they pose to the victim.

7 *Correct answer A*: This fits closely over the mouth and nose and must be breathed through, so aerosol spray becomes trapped on its outer surface rather than being inhaled. Visors do not fit closely over the mouth and nose, so aerosol contamination can still be inhaled when they are used without a face mask beneath.

8 *Correct answer B*: These materials are certainly not infectious as they are unused products that have not come into contact with patients. Offensive waste is that which is also non-infectious but which may cause offence to those who handle it – such as toilet hygiene waste and paper cleaning products that have not come into contact with body fluids.

9 *Correct answer A*: Cleaning removes any visible debris from the surface of the items, so that their whole surface is then exposed to the rest of the reprocessing procedures. Disinfection is carried out to remove some microorganisms and make the items less contaminated for handling; inspection is carried out to ensure no further visible debris remains, which could harbour other microorganisms; and then sterilisation is carried out to kill any remaining microorganisms and spores so that the items are safe for reuse.

10 *Correct answer A*: The flush stage is an initial low-temperature pressure rinse that removes gross solid and liquid debris from the items so that their surfaces are fully exposed to the succeeding stages of the cycle. The items are then washed and rinsed and undergo a higher-temperature thermal disinfection stage before being dried at the end of the cycle.

11 *Correct answer B*: Lead is no longer considered as hazardous waste in its solid form, as it was previously when it had to be disposed of as special waste. It is now only considered harmful in its liquid state, and this is not relevant in the dental workplace. Although now classed as non-hazardous waste, it must still be disposed of by a registered commercial waste handler.

12 *Correct answer B*: This is a specific test to ensure that protein is being effectively removed from items while immersed in the ultrasonic bath during a cycle. It relies not just on the ultrasonic vibration to remove solid debris but also the enzyme-based detergent that is used in solution within the bath to remove any protein residue. Test strips with special holders are available for immersion in the bath to carry out the test. Protein is present in body tissues and fluids, as well as within the structure of microorganisms.

13 *Correct answer B*: This stage of a risk assessment studies the significance of the subject in its potential to cause harm to someone; so, for example, if access to the subject is limited to certain persons only, the risk is less than if everyone has access. The risk of potential injury is considered in relation to the frequency of use of the subject, how serious an injury could be and who may be harmed – it is evaluated.

14 *Correct answer C*: Although some patients (and staff) have developed a hyper-sensitivity to latex (or even an allergy to it), latex gloves are still widely available from dental and medical suppliers and are used in many hospital and clinical environments. Powdered gloves may also produce hypersensitivity reactions, and their use is not recommended routinely, but should be limited to the occasional full surgical procedures that may be carried out in the dental workplace, where thorough hand drying after washing is not carried out before gloves are placed. The powder then absorbs the moisture remaining on the hands from inside the gloves.

15 *Correct answer C*: No type of autoclave is capable of sterilising items that have not been fully decontaminated first; if this were possible, then the whole process of decontamination would be pointless and would not need to be carried out before each cycle so scrupulously. All three of the other options are true.

16 *Correct answer D*: RIDDOR is the acronym for Reporting of Injuries, Diseases and Dangerous Occurrences Regulations – and one of the dangerous occurrences it covers is the explosion of pressure vessels, such as autoclaves. COSHH is concerned with the safe use of chemicals, HTM 01-05 with infection control in primary health-care environments, and IR(ME)R with ionising radiation regulations.

17 *Correct answer A*: The tooth is classed as a body part and is therefore catego-rised as infectious (clinical) waste. If an amalgam filling was present in the tooth, the chemical hazard of the mercury content of the filling would take precedence so that the tooth was not sent for incineration, and the correct answer would then be non-infectious waste (answer C).

18 *Correct answer C*: The contents of the machine undergo a low-temperature flush to remove gross debris particles and then are washed and rinsed. Thermal disinfection is then carried out at a higher temperature before the items are dried. On removal from the washer–disinfector, the items can then be sterilised in an autoclave.

19 *Correct answer C*: This information must be held in the infection control policy as this is the obvious place that would be searched by staff to discover the protocol to be followed in the event of such an injury. The information must be updated whenever necessary so that it is always current.

20 *Correct answer C*: Heavy-duty household gloves are recommended to be worn while contaminated instruments are being handled to avoid the possibility of a sharps injury. All three of the other options are advisable.

21 *Correct answer D*: Debris removal by cleaning and disinfection to remove some microorganism contamination are carried out initially so that all surfaces of the reusable items are able to be inspected and declared clear of any visible contamination. Only then can the items be sterilised and rendered aseptic (free from all microorganisms and spores).

22 *Correct answer A*: The risk cannot be controlled if it has not been identified and evaluated to determine what risk it poses and to whom.

23 *Correct answer B*: The ideal place for un-bagged storage for these items is within cupboards or drawers in the decontamination room itself, as this is away from all sources of contamination (the clinical area and the patients) and is therefore the cleanest room on the premises.

24 *Correct answer B*: This ensures that the door seal has no debris stuck on it, nor any wear and tear evidence, which would prevent full sealing of the chamber during a sterilisation cycle. It only needs to be carried out on a weekly basis. All three of the other options are tests or actions that must be carried out on a daily basis, rather than weekly.

25 *Correct answer D*: RIDDOR is the acronym for Reporting of Injuries, Diseases and Dangerous Occurrences Regulations – and one of the notifiable diseases that must be reported under its regulations is Legionnaires' disease. COSHH is concerned with the safe use of chemicals on the premises, and both the Environmental Protection Act and Hazardous Waste Regulations are concerned with the correct segregation and disposal of waste produced in the dental workplace.

OUTCOME 1

Understand the Various Methods of Dental Assessment

Questions

1 Which type of dental probe is specifically used to detect interproximal caries?
   A BPE probe
   B Briault probe
   C Right angle probe
   D WHO probe

2 During an oral health assessment, a patient is diagnosed with chronic gingivitis. Which one of the following is most likely to have been found when this condition is present?
   A Furcation lesions
   B Gingival hyperplasia
   C Subgingival calculus
   D True pockets

3 What is the FDI notation of the tooth charted as lower left first deciduous molar in the Palmer charting system?
   A 36
   B 47
   C 63
   D 74

4 Which one of the following radiograph views is particularly useful when a posterior tooth is suspected of having recurrent caries?
   A Anterior occlusal
   B Dental pantomograph
   C Horizontal bitewing
   D Periapical

Questions and Answers for Diploma in Dental Nursing, Level 3, First Edition. Carole Hollins.
© 2016 John Wiley & Sons, Ltd. Published 2016 by John Wiley & Sons, Ltd.

5 During an oral health assessment, the dentist will inspect various tissues of the head and neck of a patient. Which one of the following options is the tissue where squamous cell carcinoma is most likely to be seen?

A Deciduous teeth

B Floor of the mouth

C Gingiva

D Lymph nodes

6 Which one of the following terms is used to describe the type of tooth tissue loss caused by tooth grinding?

A Abrasion

B Attrition

C Caries

D Erosion

7 During an oral health assessment, a periodontal code 1 is recorded in the upper anterior sextant. Which one of the following findings does this code indicate to be present?

A Bleeding on probing

B Furcation involvement

C Plaque retention factor

D Tooth mobility

8 During an oral health assessment, the dentist may detect the presence of a periodontal pocket. Which of the following assessment methods can be used to indicate the presence of a pocket?

A Use of bitewing radiographs

B Use of BPE probe

C Use of disclosing tablets

D Use of transillumination

9 Which one of the following materials is used in a vitality test to stimulate a tooth to react to cold?

A Alginate

B Ethyl chloride

C Gutta-percha

D Sodium hypochlorite

10 Which one of the following cannot be diagnosed by the use of dental radiographs?

A Congenital tooth absence

B Dental abscess

C Jaw fracture

D Tooth vitality

11 During an oral health assessment, it is recorded that a lower second molar tooth is 'grade III mobile'. Which one of the following options does this grade indicate?

A Ankylosed tooth

B Side-to-side movement less than 2 mm

C Side-to-side movement more than 2 mm

D Vertical tooth movement

12 Which one of the following radiograph views is that most likely to be used to determine the presence of an unerupted lateral incisor?

A Anterior occlusal

B Dental pantomograph

C Horizontal bitewing

D Lateral oblique

13 During a periodontal assessment, a BPE charting is carried out. Which one of the following findings specifically indicates a BPE score 3?

A Bleeding on probing

B Furcation involvement

C Pocket depth up to 5.5 mm

D Presence of calculus

14 Various materials are used by the dental team during an oral health assessment. Which one of the following materials is used to take impressions for study models?

A Calcium and alginate salts with water

B Calcium sulphate and water

C Hardened calcium sulphate and water

D Ethyl chloride

15 Which one of the following Palmer charting notations indicates the tooth charted as 42 in the FDI charting system?

A Lower right deciduous first molar

B Lower right permanent lateral incisor

C Upper left deciduous first molar

D Upper left first premolar

16 Vitality testing is often carried out by the dentist to diagnose the source of dental pain. What is the main disadvantage to the patient during the testing?

A All tests are expensive

B All tests are time-consuming

C All tests involve a painful stimulus

D All tests may be inaccurate

17 Which one of the following terms is used to describe the type of tooth tissue loss caused by an excessive intake of dietary acids?

  A Abrasion

  B Attrition

  C Caries

  D Erosion

18 Legislation is in place to ensure that the details within medical and dental records are not disclosed to a third party, so that their contents remain confidential to the patient. The public disclosure of health records on request from a third party is excluded from which of the following acts?

  A Access to Health Records Act 1990

  B Data Protection Act 1998

  C Freedom of Information Act 2000

  D Police and Criminal Evidence Act 1984

19 Ideally, patient records should be kept indefinitely, but legally, those for a child patient who has left the practice need to be kept until the patient reaches what age?

  A 16 years old

  B 18 years old

  C 21 years old

  D 25 years old

20 What is the term used to describe the quality assurance process in place to standardise NHS record-keeping and confidentiality issues?

  A Clinical governance

  B HTM 01-05

  C Information governance

  D NICE guidelines

21 Before a patient undergoes a course of dental treatment, they must be given certain information so that they can give a valid consent. Which one of the following options is not necessary for consent to be valid?

  A Agreed in writing

  B Detail all likely costs

  C Given voluntarily

  D Specific to the treatment

22 Which one of the following is a valid example of a reason to disclose patient information to a third party without the patient's consent?

  A Confirmation of treatment to an employer

  B Requested by a spouse

    C Requested by another practice

    D Unpaid dental charges

23 Patients have a right to complain if they feel the service or treatment they have received is inadequate. Which one of the following options must the dental workplace follow in order to handle the complaint correctly?

    A Accept liability

    B Apologise unreservedly

    C Give the name of the staff member involved

    D Report back to the patient within 10 days

24 Patients have the right of access to their own health records written after 1991. Which one of the following points must all parties abide by to comply with an access request from a patient?

    A Access approved by the record holder

    B Issue a receipt

    C Release records to a family member

    D Respond to a verbal request

Answers

1 *Correct answer B*: This probe has both end tips angled so that the interproximal areas can be accessed – one angled for mesial probing and the other for distal probing. With posterior teeth, it is often the only instrument possible for accessing these areas during an oral health assessment. The BPE and WHO probes are used during periodontal assessment.

2 *Correct answer B*: Swollen gingivae are present when a patient has gingivitis (inflammation of the gums). All three of the other options are signs that are likely to be present when a patient has periodontitis, not gingivitis.

3 *Correct answer D*: In the FDI system, the lower left quadrant of deciduous teeth is denoted 7, and the first deciduous molar is tooth number 4, so the FDI notation of this tooth is 74. 36 is the lower left first permanent molar, 47 is the lower right second permanent molar, and 63 is the upper left deciduous canine tooth.

4 *Correct answer C*: The horizontal bitewing view is the best one to take of posterior teeth suspected of having recurrent caries as well as interproximal lesions. The dental pantomograph may give the same result but expose a patient to an unnecessarily large amount of radiation when viewing just a few teeth. The anterior occlusal is not suitable to view posterior teeth, and a periapical view is more suited when the roots of a tooth are under investigation.

5 *Correct answer B*: This is one of the most common areas where squamous cell carcinomas are found, as well as the underside and sides of the tongue. The condition does not affect the teeth, and other types of cancer are associated with the lymph nodes. The gingivae are only likely to be affected as the initial malignant tumour spreads if left untreated.

6 *Correct answer B*: Attrition is classically seen as a loss of the biting surface of the teeth (incisal edges and occlusal surfaces) brought about by the clenching and grinding habits of the patient. Abrasion is the tooth surface loss seen at the necks of the teeth due to overzealous toothbrushing, caries is caused by the actions of certain bacteria found in dental plaque, and erosion is enamel loss due to the action of dietary acids on the teeth.

7 *Correct answer A*: This distinguishes between fully healthy gingivae and early gingivitis. Furcation involvement occurs with BPE codes of *, the presence of plaque retention factors will be recorded as BPE 2, and tooth mobility occurs when there has been substantial bone loss around a tooth.

8 *Correct answer B*: This specially designed probe is gently inserted into the periodontal pocket so that its depth can be read off the scale marked along its length. Bitewing radiographs and transillumination are methods of detecting posterior and anterior caries, respectively, and disclosing tablets are used to stain dental plaque to assist in oral hygiene instruction and cleaning methods.

9 *Correct answer B*: Ethyl chloride is a liquid that vaporises quickly at room temperature, leaving ice crystals that provide a cold stimulus when applied to the dry surface of a tooth, especially one that is hypersensitive. Gutta-percha (as greenstick compound) is a material that can be heated and applied carefully to the teeth to provide a hot stimulus under similar circumstances. The other two options are not used for testing the vitality of teeth.

10 *Correct answer D*: This is diagnosed by the tooth's response to sensation, rather than by its appearance on a radiograph, although a tooth showing signs of an acute periapical lesion on a radiograph is likely to be dying or dead. All three of the other options can be diagnosed on a radiograph.

11 *Correct answer D*: This is the worst level of tooth mobility, where a tooth can be lifted up and down in its socket due to severe bone loss around its root or roots. Side-to-side movement of less than 2 mm is class I mobility, and that of more than 2 mm is class II mobility. An ankylosed tooth is one that is rigid in its socket, with no possible movement whatsoever.

12 *Correct answer A*: An anterior occlusal view can be taken of either the maxilla or mandible and shows the anterior six teeth (canine to canine) in full, as well as the surrounding bone of the jaw. Any of these teeth that is unerupted will also be visible on the radiograph, revealing its position in relation to the other teeth. A dental pantomograph will also reveal the presence of an unerupted tooth but less clearly than is likely with the anterior occlusal view, and the other two options are unsuitable views for this purpose.

13 *Correct answer C*: If a pocket is deeper than 5.5 mm, the BPE score would be 4, the presence of calculus as a plaque retention factor would be BPE score 2, and bleeding on probing would be BPE score 1.

14 *Correct answer A*: These are the constituents of alginate impression material that is used to take impressions for study models. Calcium sulphate and water are the constituents of dental plaster that is used to base the study models, and hardened calcium sulphate and water are the constituents of dental stone that is used to produce the yellow-coloured study model casts themselves. Ethyl chloride is a liquid used to test the vitality of a tooth.

15 *Correct answer B*: The lower right permanent dentition quadrant is 4 and the permanent lateral incisor is tooth 2, so 42 is the lower right permanent lateral incisor. The lower right deciduous first molar is FDI notation 84, the upper left deciduous first molar is FDI notation 64, and the upper left first premolar is FDI notation 24.

16 *Correct answer C*: A vital tooth will experience a sharp temperature change or an electrical stimulus, all of which are uncomfortable to the patient, if not painful. The tests are quick and inexpensive and relatively accurate with regard to identifying a hypersensitive or a dead tooth.

17 *Correct answer D*: The dietary acids found in fizzy drinks and some fruit juices, acidic fruits and foods such as pickled onions and alcoholic drinks such as wines cause demineralisation of the surface of the tooth enamel. The top layer of the enamel is softened and stripped from the tooth so that the underlying dentine layer becomes exposed, making the teeth very sensitive to especially cold stimulation. Caries is caused by the action of bacterial plaque microorganisms, abrasion is caused by overzealous toothbrushing, and attrition is caused by grinding the teeth together.

18 *Correct answer C*: Most government-held information is accessible to anyone upon request through the Freedom of Information Act 2000, but health records are specifically excluded from this legislation. The Access to Health Records Act allows a patient access to their own records upon written request, while the Police and Criminal Evidence Act allows health records to be released when requested by court order and without the patient's consent. The Data Protection Act ensures that the data controller only releases information to third parties in accordance with the conditions of the act, but some information may therefore be released.

19 *Correct answer D*: Written records cannot realistically be kept indefinitely as they would take up a considerable amount of space, while computer backup systems tend to overwrite themselves on a rolling basis unless the whole system is periodically stored to an external hard drive device, which would then have to have a large enough memory to be sufficient. Legally, therefore, a timeline is in place beyond which records can be destroyed by shredding and incineration.

20 *Correct answer C*: This has been implemented for NHS records and confidentiality issues to ensure the security and appropriate use of personal and patient information within health-care premises, including dental workplaces. It brings together all of the legal rules, information and guidance on best practice that apply to handling of patient information. All NHS workplaces are required to comply with it.

21 *Correct answer A*: This is advised routinely but oral consent is acceptable for minimal treatment, such as an oral health assessment or a simple scale and polish. The patient must always be informed of any likely costs before they agree to treatment, especially where variable treatment options are possible. The patient must never be coerced or bullied into a course of treatment or into having one option over another. The consent given must be specific to the treatment they are to receive for each course after all of the necessary information has been given for the patient to make a decision.

22 *Correct answer D*: When treatment has been provided in good faith by the dental workplace, but has then not been paid for upon request by the patient, their details can be disclosed to a debt collection service for the recovery of the debt and without the patient's consent. An employer or a spouse has no right of access to any patient information without their consent, nor does another dental practice.

23 *Correct answer D*: The time frames that must be followed at various stages of the complaints process are set down in the complaints procedure and must be followed. It is not acceptable for each stage to be dragged out as long as possible, as used to happen. Liability should never be accepted until it has been proven that the workplace was at fault, and an unreserved apology should also not be given as this implies guilt where there may be none. Names of individual staff members should not be released to the patient as they may then be personally targeted by the patient.

24 *Correct answer A*: Only the record holder (usually the dentist) can approve a patient's access to their own health records. Copies rather than originals will be released, so a receipt is not necessary although a note should be made that the records have been released in accordance with the request. The records must only be given to the patient themselves (not a family member), and the request has to be made in writing to comply with the law, so a verbal request must not be acted upon.

Assessment of Oral Health and Treatment Planning

OUTCOME 2

Know the Clinical Assessments Associated with Orthodontics

Questions

1 What is the correct term used to describe the horizontal distance between the upper and lower incisors, which is usually measured during an orthodontic assessment?
   A Anterior open bite
   B Crossbite
   C Overbite
   D Overjet

2 A 15-year-old patient is assessed as requiring orthodontic treatment for severe crowding in both arches. Which one of the following radiograph views is most likely to be required before treatment begins?
   A Dental pantomograph
   B Lateral oblique
   C Periapical
   D Vertical bitewing

3 A patient is classified as having an Angle's class II division 1 malocclusion. Which one of the following features is most likely to be present?
   A Bilateral crossbite
   B Proclined upper incisors
   C Retroclined lower incisors
   D Reverse overjet

Questions and Answers for Diploma in Dental Nursing, Level 3, First Edition. Carole Hollins.
© 2016 John Wiley & Sons, Ltd. Published 2016 by John Wiley & Sons, Ltd.

4 Which one of the following options indicates the type of orthodontic device that specifically uses the oral musculature to allow controlled movement of the mandible?

A Fixed appliance

B Fixed retainer

C Functional appliance

D Removable appliance

5 Ideal occlusion is referred to as Angle's class I and will exhibit which of the following measurements at orthodontic assessment?

A Overjet 1–2 mm, overbite 25%

B Overjet 2–3 mm, overbite 40%

C Overjet 2–4 mm, overbite 50%

D Overjet 3–5 mm, overbite 75%

6 When a patient has been accepted for orthodontic treatment at the dental workplace, which one of the following options must be discussed with ALL patients when preoperative advice is to be given?

A Need for extractions

B Need for fixed appliances

C Need for impressions

D Need for surgery

7 During an orthodontic assessment of a patient, the severity of any malocclusion present is recorded as an Index of Orthodontic Treatment Needs (IOTN) score. Which one of the following scores indicates the most severe form of malocclusion?

A IOTN 3a

B IOTN 3d

C IOTN 5a

D IOTN 5d

8 Orthodontic appliances may be removable, functional or fixed in type. Which one of the following tooth movements usually requires a fixed appliance to achieve it?

A Correction of crossbite

B Derotation

C Distal movement along the arch

D Reduction of overbite

9 Which one of the following items is used during orthodontic treatment with a removable appliance?

A Bracket

B Crib

C Molar band

D Tube

10 Which oral health product should be recommended to a patient who has had a fixed orthodontic appliance fitted to assist with cleaning beneath the archwire?

A Floss

B Interdental brush

C Mouthwash

D Toothbrush

11 Crowding occurs in dental arches when there is insufficient room in the arch to accommodate the permanent teeth. Which are the likeliest teeth to be crowded out of the upper arch?

A Canines

B First premolars

C Lateral incisors

D Second premolars

12 When setting up the surgery for an orthodontic fixed appliance fit appointment, which one of the following items must the dental nurse set out to assist in the completion of the procedure?

A Adams pliers

B Bracket holders

C Measuring ruler

D Straight handpiece

13 A patient has been classified as having a class III malocclusion. Which one of the following features is most likely to be present?

A Labial crowding

B Proclined upper incisors

C Reverse overjet

D Unilateral crossbite

14 What is the correct term used to describe the vertical distance between the upper and lower incisors, which is usually measured during an orthodontic assessment?

A Anterior open bite

B Crossbite

C Overbite

D Overjet

15 Which one of the following oral health products should be recommended to fixed orthodontic patients specifically to reduce the likelihood of enamel decalcification during treatment?

A Dental floss

B Electric toothbrush

C Fluoride mouthwash

D Interdental brush

16 The classification of malocclusion may be determined by the relative positions of the first molar teeth to each other between the arches. When the mesiobuccal cusp of the upper molar lies behind the buccal groove of the lower molar, which one of the following classifications is present?

A Class I

B Class II division 1

C Class II division 2

D Class III

17 When setting up the surgery for a functional appliance adjustment appointment, which item is required to tighten the appliance?

A Adams pliers

B Alastik holders

C Band removers

D End cutters

18 What material is normally used to construct palatal finger springs that will be incorporated into a removable orthodontic appliance?

A Acrylic

B Cobalt chrome

C Nickel titanium

D Stainless steel

Answers

1 *Correct answer D*: This measurement is taken horizontally from the incisal edge of the upper incisors to the labial surface of the lower incisors with a ruler. A class I occlusion will measure 2–4 mm, and this will usually be increased in class II cases (especially class II division 1 cases) and reduced in class III cases.

2 *Correct answer A*: A dental pantomograph should always be taken before starting orthodontic treatment to screen the patient for healthy teeth and jaw bones and to check for unexpected findings such as a supernumerary tooth or other pathology.

3 *Correct answer B*: Proclined upper incisors are the distinguishing feature of most class II division 1 cases. The lower jaw is too far back so that the upper incisors escape the confines of the lower lip and become trapped outside it, so that they are held in a prominent proclined position.

4 *Correct answer C*: Functional appliances are designed to hold the jaws in a class I occlusion when they are worn correctly, so that the oral musculature develops into this position gradually as growth occurs. This results in a stable class I occlusion at the end of treatment. The same result can be achieved with a fixed appliance and traction, but the fixed appliance is not designed specifically to achieve this.

5 *Correct answer C*: An overjet less than 2 mm suggests a tendency to class III in most cases, and larger than 4 mm a tendency to class II. Deep overbites of more than 50% are often found in class II division 2 cases, while reduced overbites of less than 50% are often seen in class III cases.

6 *Correct answer C*: All orthodontic patients must have pre- and post-treatment study models taken, without exception, as these provide a record of the treatment result. Impressions will also be required to make removable and functional appliances and for retainers to be made at the end of treatment.

7 *Correct answer C*: The higher the number, the more severe the case, so score 5 is the most severe. The closer the letter to 'a', the more severe the orthodontic feature that is present, so IOTN score 5a is the most severe, and indicates a patient with an increased overjet of more than 9 mm.

8 *Correct answer B*: Often, the most difficult movement to achieve (and the most likely to relapse) is the derotation of a twisted tooth. The anchorage of a fixed appliance provides sufficient force to achieve this movement without dislodging the brackets from the teeth, but the same cannot be achieved with removable or functional appliances.

9 *Correct answer B*: The Adams crib is the retention feature of removable appliances. They are usually placed onto molar and premolar teeth and can be tightened at each appointment to maintain the fit of the appliance during treatment. All three of the other options are features of a fixed appliance.

10 *Correct answer B*: These are recommended for particular cleaning beneath an archwire, as the heads are small and can be bent in various directions to assist cleaning. Ordinary toothbrushes are too large to clean beneath the archwire, and floss cannot be used when the archwire is in place. The use of mouthwash will also be recommended during treatment, but not specifically for cleaning beneath the archwire.

11 *Correct answer A*: Upper canines are usually the last teeth to erupt except for the second and third molars, and their position at the 'corners' of the dental arch make them most likely to be pushed out of line during their late eruption. They then tend to be forced buccally and erupt as prominent 'fangs' or they become impacted in the palate in a position palatal to the arch.

12 *Correct answer B*: As the name suggests, these are used to hold individual brackets while they are positioned onto individual teeth during the bonding procedure. Adams pliers and a straight handpiece are required for removable appliances, and a measuring ruler is used for taking overjet measurements before, during and after treatment.

13 *Correct answer C*: A reverse overjet is a feature of many class III cases, where the lower jaw is further forward than normal so that the overjet is reduced below 2 mm, or the teeth bite edge to edge, or the lower jaw is so far forwards that the upper incisors lie behind the lower incisors and there is a reverse (negative) overjet.

14 *Correct answer C*: Normally, the upper incisors overlap the lower incisors vertically and cover about 50% of the surface of the lower incisors in class I cases. This is called the overbite. In class II division 2 cases, the overbite can be as great as 100% (deep overbite), and in class III cases, the overbite is often reduced below 50% or is recorded as 0% when the teeth bite edge to edge, or there is no overbite when the teeth do not touch – this is called an anterior open bite.

15 *Correct answer C*: Fluoride mouthwash supplies additional fluoride for the teeth to incorporate into their enamel structure during fixed orthodontic treatment, over and above that supplied by fluoride toothpaste. As a mouthwash, the fluoride will be more accessible to all tooth areas and can be taken up to repair areas of decalcification or to prevent decalcification occurring by strengthening the enamel surface and making it more resistant to acid attack. It is recommended particularly in fixed appliance cases because adequate cleaning of these devices and the teeth beneath them requires huge effort by the patient, and the mouthwash assists them greatly.

16 *Correct answer D*: The upper mesiobuccal cusp should lie in the lower mesiobuccal groove in class I cases, so if it lies behind this position, then the lower jaw is too far forwards. This is a feature of class III cases.

17 *Correct answer A*: Functional appliances rely for their retention on Adams cribs, the same as removable appliances, and these are adjusted using the Adams pliers. All three of the other options are instruments required for use on a fixed appliance.

18 *Correct answer D*: The stainless steel used is thinner than for Adams cribs so that it is more flexible and easily adjusted during treatment but is still strong enough to hold its position around the tooth. Cobalt chrome is too stiff to be adjusted in this way, nickel titanium is used in archwires during fixed appliance treatment, and acrylic is the plastic material used to construct the base plates of removable and functional appliances and some retainers.

OUTCOME 3
Understand the Changes That May Occur in the Oral Tissues

Questions

1 Which one of the following diseases of the oral soft tissues is associated with infection by bacteria?
   A Herpes simplex
   B Oral candidiasis
   C Periodontitis
   D Stomatitis

2 Which one of the following diseases of the oral mucosa is described as the presence of several small, shallow, painful ulcers that heal to leave no scarring?
   A Herpetiform ulceration
   B Major aphthous ulceration
   C Minor aphthous ulceration
   D Squamous cell carcinoma

3 Which one of the following oral soft tissue diseases is most likely to occur after a patient has taken a long course of broad-spectrum antibiotics?
   A Herpes simplex
   B Herpetiform aphthous ulcers
   C Leukoplakia
   D Oral candidiasis

4 A patient presenting with an inflamed tongue that appears smooth and red may be deficient in which one of the following?
   A Fluoride
   B Gluten
   C Iron
   D Vitamin C

Questions and Answers for Diploma in Dental Nursing, Level 3, First Edition. Carole Hollins.
© 2016 John Wiley & Sons, Ltd. Published 2016 by John Wiley & Sons, Ltd.

5 Which one of the following diseases of the oral mucosa is NOT classed as an inflammatory condition?

   A Angular cheilitis

   B Erythroplakia

   C Glossitis

   D Stomatitis

6 Which one of the following is an effect that often occurs in older patients due to age-related changes to their teeth?

   A Decreased tooth sensitivity

   B Occlusal caries

   C Root curvature

   D Whitened teeth

7 The dental specialism of managing the specific oral health care of elderly patients is known by which one of the following terms?

   A Gerodontics

   B Orthodontics

   C Paedodontics

   D Prosthodontics

8 Various medical conditions may affect the oral tissues detrimentally. Which one of the following effects is often seen in patients who are diagnosed with type 2 diabetes?

   A Aphthous ulcers

   B Enamel erosion

   C Poor wound healing

   D Stomatitis

9 Various age-related changes occur to the body tissues, including those of the oral cavity. Which one of the following tissues is most likely to be affected when osteoporosis develops?

   A Bone

   B Oral mucosa

   C Salivary glands

   D Skin

10 Which one of the following diseases of the oral mucosa is described as an immovable white patch that has no obvious cause?

   A Leukoplakia

   B Major aphthous ulceration

   C Oral candidiasis

   D Squamous cell carcinoma

11 Which one of the following oral conditions may be seen in a patient who suffers from gastric reflux?

A Attrition

B Erosion

C Glossitis

D Xerostomia

12 Which one of the following inflammatory disorders affecting the oral cavity is often determined as being psychogenic in origin?

A Angular cheilitis

B Burning mouth syndrome

C Erythroplakia

D Hand, foot and mouth disease

13 Which one of the following conditions is not related to age and therefore is not likely to occur more frequently as a patient ages?

A Osteoporosis

B Periapical abscess

C Root caries

D Xerostomia

14 Which one of the following oral diseases can be seen as a painless ulcer with no obvious cause and which fails to fully heal within three weeks of dental intervention?

A Chronic periapical abscess

B Herpes simplex type 1

C Major aphthous ulceration

D Squamous cell carcinoma

15 Which one of the following conditions is linked specifically to acquired immune deficiency syndrome (AIDS)?

A Kaposi's sarcoma

B Leukoplakia

C Oral candidiasis

D Squamous cell carcinoma

16 Patients who suffer from coeliac disease have an intolerance to the cereal protein gluten. Which one of the following oral lesions is not usually found in these patients?

A Glossitis

B Stomatitis

C Ulceration

D Xerostomia

17 The herpes group of viruses can affect the oral soft tissues in a variety of ways. Which virus is responsible for the lesion known as a 'cold sore'?

   A Herpes labialis

   B Herpes simplex

   C Herpes varicella

   D Herpes zoster

18 Erosion is the non-carious loss of tooth enamel due to damage by extrinsic acids. Which one of the following medical conditions is most likely to be linked to tooth erosion?

   A Bulimia

   B Coeliac disease

   C Diabetes

   D Epilepsy

Answers

1 *Correct answer C*: Various bacteria are associated with periodontal disease, in particular *Actinomyces* and *Treponema* species, as well as specific microorganisms such as *Porphyromonas gingivalis*. Herpes simplex is caused by the virus of the same name, and both oral candidiasis and stomatitis are caused by fungal infection with *Candida albicans*.

2 *Correct answer C*: These are commonly seen in some patients' mouths and are associated with stress and certain metabolic deficiencies. Major aphthous ulcers are larger and tend to scar on healing. Herpetiform ulceration usually occurs in huge numbers of tiny ulcers – up to a hundred at a time. Squamous cell carcinomas do not heal but gradually increase in size and are usually painless initially – these are the sinister signs that should prompt a referral to the hospital.

3 *Correct answer D*: Broad-spectrum antibiotics are not exclusive to the bacteria they act against, and very often, their prolonged use will result in the death of harmless bacteria that are normally present in the patient's body (commensal bacteria), as well as the pathogens for which they were originally prescribed. The fungus *C. albicans* will then take advantage of this situation of low bacteria levels and will grow and set up its own colonies of microorganisms. It is referred to in these situations as an opportunistic pathogen. The presence of any of the three other options is not associated with courses of antibiotics.

4 *Correct answer C*: The condition described is glossitis – inflammation of the tongue. It is often seen in iron deficiency anaemia cases and may also indicate vitamin B deficiency. The condition has no association with any of the three other options.

5 *Correct answer B*: This is a red patch on the oral mucosa of unknown cause and is considered to be a premalignant lesion that requires hospital investigation. As a rule of thumb, any condition with the suffix '-itis' indicates an inflammatory condition (e.g. pulpitis, gingivitis, appendicitis, periodontitis and so on). All three of the other options are therefore inflammatory conditions.

6 *Correct answer A*: The pulp chambers narrow with age, and teeth tend to become less sensitive in older patients; indeed, the lack of pain they can experience with fractured or infected teeth is often surprising. There is no relationship with increased age and caries incidence. Roots are formed during tooth development in childhood and do not change with time. Teeth tend to darken with age, rather than become lighter.

7 *Correct answer A*: The study of dental issues in elderly patients is called gerodontology. Orthodontics is the specialism concerned with the correction of malocclusions (using orthodontic appliances), paedodontics is the specialism concerned with children's oral health care, and prosthodontics is the specialism concerned with tooth replacement (crowns, bridges, dentures, implants and so on).

8 *Correct answer C*: Diabetics tend to suffer from poor peripheral circulation that causes poor wound healing. They are therefore prone to postoperative problems after surgery, are at risk of developing periodontal disease that often fails to respond to routine treatment and often develop unexpected periapical lesions that require endodontic intervention to save teeth. There is no link with diabetes and all three of the other options.

9 *Correct answer A*: This is a gradual thinning of the bone that often occurs in postmenopausal women due to the reduction of oestrogen in the body at this time. The bones become brittle as the thinning progresses and fracture more readily following trauma – this includes trauma such as tooth extraction. However, age-related osteoporosis can also occur, and in both sexes, so elderly male patients may be at risk of jaw fracture during dental surgery too. All three of the other options are not associated with changes developing at the onset of osteoporosis.

10 *Correct answer A*: Leukoplakia is regarded as a potentially premalignant condition and is particularly associated with smoking and heavy alcohol intake. Patients presenting with Leukoplakia and these social issues should be referred for further investigation. Oral candidiasis can be diagnosed by the ability to wipe the white patch off the mucosa to leave a red area beneath.

11 *Correct answer B*: Acidic stomach contents will be regurgitated in these patients, causing enamel erosion over time. Attrition is the enamel loss caused by tooth grinding and affects the occlusal surfaces and incisal edges of the teeth. Glossitis is the inflammation of the tongue and is often seen in patients with an underlying medical condition. Xerostomia is a persistently reduced salivary flow causing a dry mouth and is usually due to age-related changes or disease of the salivary glands.

12 *Correct answer B*: A condition regarded as having no physical basis (so no abnormality or disease is diagnosed) and therefore is considered to be 'of the mind'. It is often determined that the sufferer has a genuine anxiety regarding a fear of developing cancer or other serious illness, or is depressed.

13 *Correct answer B*: A periapical abscess can occur at any time of life, but is not age related. A tooth can undergo trauma or have gross caries present in a child or an elderly patient. All three of the other options are more likely to occur as a patient ages due to the natural changes that occur to the oral and body tissues as the patient grows older.

14 *Correct answer D*: These are the determining features of a lesion that should send alarm bells ringing that it may be sinister in nature and prompt an urgent referral of the patient to the hospital for specialist investigation.

15 *Correct answer A*: This is an unusual lesion that occurs in the palate (or on the skin) as a purplish brown growth and is a rare occurrence in a healthy individual but a classic development in a patient with autoimmune deficiency syndrome (AIDS). All three of the other options may occur as frequently in otherwise healthy patients as they can in AIDS sufferers.

16 *Correct answer D*: Sufferers of coeliac disease may develop various oral inflammations and ulcerations from time to time, but they do not suffer from a persistent dry mouth (xerostomia). It is not related to their medical condition.

17 *Correct answer A*: Although the primary herpes infection will have been due to herpes simplex, the virus remains in the trigeminal nerve and is referred to as herpes labialis, and this microorganism is responsible for the development of a cold sore. Herpes varicella causes chickenpox, while herpes zoster causes shingles.

18 *Correct answer A*: Bulimia is an emotional disorder in which the sufferer has bouts of compulsive overeating followed by periods of self-induced vomiting or fasting. The frequent regurgitation of the acidic stomach contents causes enamel erosion of certain teeth, in a pattern involving the palatal surfaces of the upper teeth, which indicates that the cause is frequent vomiting. They may also exhibit a burnt or reddened oropharynx, which has been produced by the frequent passage of acidic vomit.

Know the Medical Emergencies That May Occur in the Dental Environment

Questions

1 Which one of the following groups of signs would indicate that a casualty is suffering an asthma attack?
   A Breathless, cyanosis, wheezing on expiration
   B Coughing or wheezing, cyanosis
   C Facial swelling, rash, gasping
   D Trembling, drowsy, slurred speech

2 Which one of the following is the current correct ratio of chest compressions to rescue breaths that must be carried out during cardiopulmonary resuscitation on a casualty?
   A 15:1
   B 30:1
   C 15:2
   D 30:2

3 Which medical emergency is most likely to have occurred if the rescuer sees signs of a pale and clammy skin and a weak and thready pulse in the casualty?
   A Anaphylaxis
   B Angina attack
   C Faint
   D Hypoglycaemic episode

Questions and Answers for Diploma in Dental Nursing, Level 3, First Edition. Carole Hollins.
© 2016 John Wiley & Sons, Ltd. Published 2016 by John Wiley & Sons, Ltd.

4 Which one of the following signs is not likely to be seen when an adult casualty is choking?

A Gasping action

B Inability to speak

C Laboured breathing

D Red lips

5 Which one of the following medical emergency drugs may be administered to assist a casualty who is suffering an anaphylactic reaction?

A Adrenaline

B Aspirin

C Midazolam

D Salbutamol

6 Many dental workplaces have an automatic external defibrillator (AED) on the premises for use in certain medical emergency situations. Which one of the following is an event for which the AED can be used?

A Arrhythmia

B Asystole

C Valvular defect

D Ventricular fibrillation

7 The scale used to indicate the level of responsiveness of a casualty in an emergency situation is referred to as 'AVPU'. Which one of the following is the level of responsiveness indicated by 'A' in this scale?

A Able

B Alert

C Anxious

D Aware

8 Medical emergencies are correctly identified by their signs and symptoms. Which one of the following is a sign rather than a symptom?

A Dizziness

B Nausea

C Pain

D Pale skin

9 When an adult casualty suddenly begins to choke, which one of the following actions should the rescuer first carry out?

A Abdominal thrusts (Heimlich manoeuvre)

B Back slaps

C Encourage coughing

D Open the airway

10 Which of the following groups of signs would indicate that a casualty has suffered a cardiac arrest?
A Blue lips, no chest movements
B Grey pallor, no pulse, no chest movements
C Grey pallor, very weak pulse
D Purple face, gasping movements

11 The conscious sedation drug Midazolam may also be used in an oral form during a medical emergency. Which one of the following medical emergencies may require the use of this drug?
A Anaphylaxis
B Epileptic fit
C Hypoglycaemic episode
D Myocardial infarction

12 Under normal circumstances, what is the most likely cause of a cardiac arrest in a baby?
A Airway obstruction
B Drowning
C Electrocution
D Heart problem

13 Which blood vessel can become compressed in a heavily pregnant woman if resuscitation attempts are carried out with the casualty lying on her back, rather than tilted to the left?
A Aorta
B Coronary artery
C Inferior vena cava
D Pulmonary vein

14 Which one of the following groups of signs would indicate that a casualty is suffering from a severe hypoglycaemia?
A Breathless, cyanosis
B Coughing or wheezing, cyanosis
C Facial swelling, rash, gasping
D Trembling, drowsy, slurred speech

15 Which one of the following medical emergency drugs must be administered by intramuscular injection rather than orally?
A Adrenaline
B Aspirin
C Glyceryl trinitrate
D Salbutamol

16 What is the major difference between resuscitation attempts in a young child and an adult?

A Airway does not need to be opened

B Less chest compressions between rescue breaths

C More chest compressions between rescue breaths

D Rescue breathing commences before chest compressions

17 The scale used to indicate the level of responsiveness of a casualty in an emergency situation is referred to as 'AVPU'. Which one of the following is the level of responsiveness indicated by 'U' in this scale?

A Unaware

B Unresponsive

C Unsettled

D Upset

18 Medical emergencies are correctly identified by their signs and symptoms. Which one of the following is a symptom rather than a sign?

A Blue lips

B Chest pain

C Sweating

D Weak pulse

19 Which one of the following actions should the rescuer perform to aid a conscious casualty who is suffering a severe angina attack?

A Administer glucagon

B Begin cardiopulmonary resuscitation

C Lay the casualty flat

D Maintain the casualty upright

20 Which one of the following groups of signs would indicate that a casualty is suffering an anaphylactic reaction to latex?

A Breathless, cyanosis

B Coughing or wheezing, cyanosis

C Facial swelling, rash, gasping

D Trembling, drowsy, slurred speech

Answers

1 *Correct answer A*: Asthma is a hypersensitivity condition affecting the respiratory airways. On exposure to an inhaled allergen, the airways narrow so that air has to be forced out of the lungs, giving the characteristic wheezing noise on expiration. The sufferer becomes breathless and the lack of oxygen shows as cyanosis, especially of the lips (dark reddish-purple colouring).

2 *Correct answer D*: Thirty compressions at a rate of 100 per minute are sufficient to pump each volume of reoxygenated blood out of the heart and into the circulatory system. The oxygen is replenished by two rescue breaths after each compression cycle.

3 *Correct answer C*: A simple faint is the most likely medical emergency event that will occur in the dental workplace, especially due to the fear and anxiety that pending dental treatment provokes in some patients. The signs listed are classic of a simple faint.

4 *Correct answer D*: When any casualty is choking, they will be struggling to relieve a partially or fully blocked airway. Their oxygen intake will be severely reduced or absent, and this will result in cyanosis – a dark reddish-purple to blue colouring that will be particularly apparent in the lips. Red lips indicate good, rather than poor, oxygenation.

5 *Correct answer A*: Anaphylaxis is a severe allergic reaction to an allergen, where the immune system overreacts in response to the allergen, causing sudden and severe tissue swelling and a catastrophic fall in blood pressure that results in collapse. An intramuscular injection of 1:1000 adrenaline from the emergency drug kit as soon as possible is imperative if the casualty is to survive. Oral aspirin is given when a myocardial infarction is suspected, oral midazolam when a prolonged epileptic fit occurs, and a salbutamol inhaler is used to alleviate the symptoms of an asthma attack.

6 *Correct answer D*: Ventricular fibrillation is the condition where the heart is beating ineffectively, at a fast rate but in an uncoordinated rhythm – the AED is used to shock the muscle back into the correct rhythm, hence its title 'defibrillator'. Many people have an abnormal heart rhythm (an arrhythmia) and it is not a medical emergency, and other people are born with valvular defects – some require surgery to correct the defect while others go undiagnosed with no ill effects. When the heart goes into asystole, it has stopped beating completely and requires drugs to restart it. The AED will have no effect in this situation; in fact its use may compound the emergency.

7 *Correct answer B*: The AVPU scale is used as a quick method of assessing the level of responsiveness of a casualty in an emergency situation; the less they respond to stimuli, the lower their level of consciousness and the more serious the emergency. The scale is as follows: A=alert, V=responds to verbal stimuli, P=responds to painful stimuli and U=unresponsive.

8 *Correct answer D*: Signs are seen by the rescuer and symptoms are felt by the casualty. The colour of the skin can be seen by the rescuer as a sign, it cannot be felt by the casualty. All three of the other options are felt by the casualty and are therefore symptoms.

9 *Correct answer C*: Choking occurs when the airway is partially or fully blocked by an obstruction, which may be a foreign body or a swelling in the airway. The easiest method of removing a foreign body obstruction is to cough – this is the body's own protective mechanism of expelling objects from the airway. The casualty should initially be encouraged to cough (sometimes, they panic and forget to do so otherwise). If the object is not removed, then back slaps should be administered, and if these fail, then abdominal thrusts should be carried out. The airway cannot be opened while the blockage is still present.

10 *Correct answer B*: The heart has stopped beating if there is no pulse, the grey pallor and lack of chest movements indicate that there is no blood oxygenation and no respiratory effort being made by the casualty. Blue lips and no chest movements indicate a respiratory arrest as the oxygen levels in the blood have fallen dramatically when breathing efforts have stopped. A congested, purple facial appearance with gasping movements indicates an airway obstruction, as the casualty is choking.

11 *Correct answer B*: The midazolam is presented as a buccal gel that is rubbed onto the buccal soft tissues when a casualty has a prolonged epileptic fit or suffers repeated fits without a period of recovery between them. The jaws will be clamped tightly shut during the fitting episode, so the only available oral soft tissues for the rescuer to apply the drug will be the inner surfaces of the cheeks and the buccal sides of the alveolar ridges. The emergency services must still be called even if the casualty comes out of the fit.

12 *Correct answer A*: The vast majority of cardiac arrests in babies and young children are due to an airway obstruction, unlike in adults where the usual cause is a heart problem. Drowning and electrocution may well result in cardiac arrests, but they only occur in certain situations and do not form the majority of incidents involving babies.

13 *Correct answer C*: The inferior vena cava returns deoxygenated blood from the lower parts of the body to the right side of the heart, where it is pumped to the lungs for reoxygenation. As a vein, the vessel can be squashed closed, and this will happen in a heavily pregnant woman lying on her back, so that chest compressions during resuscitation attempts cannot force the blood around the body because it cannot pass through the compressed vena cava. In these situations, the casualty should be propped at an angle onto their left side, so that the blood vessel does not lie squashed beneath the weight of the foetus and rescue attempts are more likely to succeed.

14 *Correct answer D*: This medical emergency may occur in a diabetic patient who has either not followed their insulin regime correctly or has not eaten at the correct time, causing a dangerous fall in their blood glucose levels that may result in collapse. The classic signs they exhibit resemble severe drunkenness with the casualty becoming irritable and aggressive, having slurred speech and profuse sweating and becoming drowsy and unable to be roused.

15 *Correct answer A*: Adrenaline is injected as a 1:1000 solution intramuscularly during anaphylaxis and cannot be administered by an alternative route. Aspirin is given as a tablet to be chewed by a conscious casualty suffering a myocardial infarction, while glyceryl trinitrate is administered as a sublingual spray during an angina attack. Salbutamol is taken through an inhaler during an asthma attack.

16 *Correct answer D*: The likely cause of collapse in a young child is shortage of oxygen to their vital organs following an airway obstruction, so it is imperative that rescue breaths are given before chest compressions begin in these situations. There is little point in carrying out chest compressions if the child's lungs are empty of oxygen, so the rescue breaths are aimed at providing oxygen initially and then it can be pumped around the body to the vital organs, hopefully resulting in the resuscitation of the young casualty.

17 *Correct answer B*: The AVPU scale is used as a quick method of assessing the level of responsiveness of a casualty in an emergency situation; the less they respond to stimuli, the lower their level of consciousness and the more serious the emergency. The scale is as follows: A=alert, V=responds to verbal stimuli, P=responds to painful stimuli and U=unresponsive. If the casualty is assessed as 'U', then they are effectively unconscious and dependent on the rescuer to maintain their airway until they regain consciousness.

18 *Correct answer B*: Signs are seen by the rescuer and symptoms are felt by the casualty. Chest pain will be felt by the casualty but it cannot be seen by the rescuer, so it is a symptom. All three of the other options are signs that will be seen by the rescuer.

19 *Correct answer D*: Sitting upright while suffering an angina attack assists the casualty to breathe more easily during the attack, while lying them down increases the sensation of crushing in their chest and exacerbates their chest pain. Cardiopulmonary resuscitation should only be carried out on an unconscious casualty or where breathing is abnormal or absent. Glucagon is an emergency drug that is administered by intramuscular injection to a casualty who is unconscious and suffering from hypoglycaemia.

20 *Correct answer C*: Anaphylaxis is a severe allergic reaction to an allergen, such as latex. The immune system overreacts to exposure to the allergen resulting in a rapid and severe swelling of the face and neck tissues. A visible red rash will quickly develop, and the casualty will begin gasping for breath as their airway swells and closes. A rapid fall in their blood pressure will result in collapse.

OUTCOME 5

Know the Basic Structure and Function of Oral and Dental Anatomy

Questions

1 Which one of the following options shows the correct FDI charting notation for the tooth charted as the upper left deciduous canine in the Palmer system?
   A 23
   B 32
   C 36
   D 63

2 Which one of the following average age ranges shows that of the usual eruption date of the upper second permanent molars?
   A 3–4 years
   B 6–7 years
   C 9–11 years
   D 12–13 years

3 Which one of the following tooth types is only found in the secondary dentition?
   A Canines
   B First premolars
   C Lateral incisors
   D Second molars

4 Which one of the following options is the permanent tooth that can be identified as having three roots and five cusps?
   A Lower first molar
   B Lower second molar
   C Upper first molar
   D Upper second molar

Questions and Answers for Diploma in Dental Nursing, Level 3, First Edition. Carole Hollins.
© 2016 John Wiley & Sons, Ltd. Published 2016 by John Wiley & Sons, Ltd.

5 Which one of the following options states the tooth that is usually the largest of all teeth?

A Canine

B First molar

C Second premolar

D Second molar

6 Which one of the following average age ranges shows that of the usual eruption date of the lower permanent central incisors?

A 3–4 years

B 6–7 years

C 9–11 years

D 12–13 years

7 Which one of the following options shows the only tooth of the permanent dentition that has two roots and two cusps?

A Lower second molar

B Lower second premolar

C Upper first molar

D Upper first premolar

8 Which one of the following options shows the tooth that usually has the longest root of all teeth?

A Lower canine

B Lower first premolar

C Upper canine

D Upper second premolar

9 Which one of the following options describes the correct Palmer charting notation for the tooth charted as 43 in the FDI system?

A Lower left first premolar

B Lower right permanent canine

C Upper left first premolar

D Upper right permanent canine

10 Which one of the following tooth types is found in both the primary and secondary dentitions?

A First molar

B First premolar

C Second premolar

D Third molar

11 Which one of the following options is the correct term used to describe the natural shedding of deciduous teeth?

A Exfoliation

B Extraction

C Remineralisation

D Resorption

12 Which one of the following options shows the tooth that is usually the smallest of all teeth?

A Lower central incisor

B Lower lateral incisor

C Upper central incisor

D Upper lateral incisor

13 Which one of the four tissues that form all teeth is not composed of calcium hydroxyapatite crystals?

A Cementum

B Dentine

C Enamel

D Pulp

14 Which of the following options is an anatomical distinction that allows a molar tooth to be identified as deciduous rather than permanent?

A Darker colour

B Fewer cusps

C Larger pulp chamber

D Straight roots

15 Which one of the following options shows the two tissues that lie at the amelodentinal junction?

A Cementum and dentine

B Cementum and enamel

C Enamel and dentine

D Pulp and dentine

16 Which one of the following options is the correct dental term used to describe the surface of a tooth furthest away from the centre line?

A Buccal

B Distal

C Labial

D Mesial

17 Hydroxyl ions in calcium hydroxyapatite crystals can be exchanged with fluoride ions to form fluorapatite crystals. In which tissue layer of a tooth does this exchange of ions occur?

A Cementum
B Dentine
C Enamel
D Pulp

18 Which one of the following options is the correct dental term used to describe the surface of a tooth that lies against the tongue?

A Buccal
B Labial
C Lingual
D Palatal

19 When a tooth is extracted, the periodontal ligament fibres must be severed to allow the tooth to be removed from the socket. Which type of fibre form the majority that must be severed during this procedure?

A Alveolar crest fibres
B Apical fibres
C Oblique fibres
D Transeptal fibres

20 Which one of the following options is the tooth tissue that has collagen fibres from the periodontal ligament inserted into its outer structure?

A Cementum
B Dentine
C Enamel
D Pulp

21 Which one of the following terms is used to describe the specialised oral soft tissue that is directly attached to a tooth?

A Attached gingiva
B Dentinocemental junction
C Junctional epithelium
D Marginal gingiva

22 Which one of the following terms is used to describe the anatomical mechanical barrier that is normally present between the oral cavity and the deeper periodontal tissues?

A Free gingival groove
B Junctional attachment
C Lamina dura
D Mucoperiosteum

23 When a patient suffers from gingivitis, their gingivae appear swollen and inflamed. Which one of the following options does this phenomena give rise to?
   A False pockets
   B Halitosis
   C Periodontal abscess
   D Tartar build-up

24 Which group of periodontal ligament fibres are responsible for maintaining a tight gingival cuff around each tooth?
   A Apical fibres
   B Free gingival fibres
   C Horizontal fibres
   D Oblique fibres

25 Saliva is made up of many different components. Which one of these components allows the neutralisation of dietary acids to take place?
   A Antibodies
   B Leucocytes
   C Minerals
   D Water

26 Which one of the following salivary glands is most likely to be affected by the viral infection known as mumps?
   A Accessory gland
   B Parotid gland
   C Sublingual gland
   D Submandibular gland

27 Saliva is made up of many different components. Which one of these components begins starch digestion in the food bolus?
   A Antibacterial enzyme
   B Calcium phosphate
   C Immunoglobulin A
   D Salivary amylase

28 Which one of the following effects is not likely to be seen in a patient suffering from xerostomia?
   A Difficulty swallowing
   B Excessive salivation
   C High caries rate
   D Poor taste sensation

29 The temporomandibular joint is formed between the mandible and the skull to allow jaw movements. Which one of the following options describes the correct bones of the jaw and the skull that form this joint?

A Coronoid process and maxilla

B Coronoid process and parietal bone

C Head of the condyle and temporal bone

D Ramus of the mandible and temporal bone

30 Which pair of muscles of mastication contract together to allow the mandible to move forwards so the teeth are in a 'tip to tip' position?

A Lateral pterygoid

B Masseter

C Medial pterygoid

D Temporalis

31 The head and neck region are innervated by the 12 pairs of cranial nerves. Which one of the following options is the pair of cranial nerves that supply the muscles of mastication?

A Facial nerve

B Glossopharyngeal nerve

C Hypoglossal nerve

D Trigeminal nerve

32 Which one of the following is the blood vessel supplying the majority of the oxygenated blood supply to the oral cavity?

A Buccal artery

B Carotid artery

C Facial artery

D Temporal artery

33 Which pair of muscles of mastication are visible around the angle of the mandible when the patient clenches their jaw?

A Lateral pterygoid

B Masseter

C Medial pterygoid

D Temporalis

34 When a patient requires the extraction of the lower right second molar tooth, which one of the combination of nerves shown must be anaesthetised before the procedure is carried out?

A Inferior dental and long buccal nerves

B Lingual, inferior dental and long buccal nerves

C Long buccal and lingual nerves

D Mental, long buccal and lingual nerves

35 Which of the salivary glands is innervated by the glossopharyngeal nerve and is most likely to be associated with tumours?

A Accessory glands

B Parotid glands

C Sublingual glands

D Submandibular glands

36 Which one of the following foramina is a feature of the mandible?

A Incisive foramen

B Infra-orbital foramen

C Lesser palatine foramen

D Mental foramen

37 What is the correct term used to describe the painful muscle contractions affecting the muscles of mastication that can prevent the mouth from being opened by the patient?

A Attrition

B Bruxism

C Subluxation

D Trismus

38 Which of the following statements about diseases affecting the oral mucosa is true?

A Cold sore lesions are caused by a bacterial infection

B Leukoplakia is considered a premalignant condition

C Patients with diabetes often have oral ulceration

D Ulcerative colitis is often linked to oral cancer

39 Localised bone death (osteonecrosis) may occur in patients suffering from which one of the following conditions?

A Osteoarthritis

B Osteoporosis

C Rheumatoid arthritis

D Xerostomia

40 Which one of the following oral lesions is caused by an infection with *Candida albicans*?

A Aphthous ulcers

B Cold sore

C Denture stomatitis

D Leukoplakia

41 Which one of the following terms is used to describe a shallow break in the
oral mucosa that leaves a raw and painful circular lesion?
   A Cyst
   B Leucoplakia
   C Tumour
   D Ulcer

42 Which one of the following conditions that may affect the oral soft tissues is
not considered to be premalignant?
   A Erythroplakia
   B Leukoplakia
   C Lichen planus
   D Major aphthous ulcers

Answers

1 *Correct answer D*: The upper left deciduous quadrant is charted as 6, and the canine tooth as 3, so this tooth is 63 in the FDI system. Tooth 23 is the upper left permanent canine, 32 is the lower left permanent lateral incisor, and 36 is the lower left permanent first molar.

2 *Correct answer D*: The second permanent molars are usually the last teeth to erupt except for the wisdom teeth, if the patient has any. No permanent teeth erupt at 3–4 years of age, the first ones being the first permanent molars and the lower central incisors at 6–7 years of age. The first premolars begin erupting between 9 and 11 years of age.

3 *Correct answer B*: There are no premolars in the primary dentition. The first and second premolars of the secondary dentition are preceded by the first and second primary molars, respectively. All three of the other options are present in both the primary and secondary dentitions.

4 *Correct answer C*: Only the upper molar teeth have three roots, and only the first molars in both arches have five cusps. The fifth cusp of the upper first molar is often small and positioned on the palatal wall of the tooth and is called the cusp of Carabelli.

5 *Correct answer B*: The molar teeth in both arches are the largest, and the first molars have five cusps, while the others only have four. The first molars are therefore the largest of the teeth.

6 *Correct answer B*: These are the first of the permanent teeth to erupt, along with the first permanent molars at about the same time. No permanent teeth erupt at 3–4 years of age, the first premolars begin erupting at around 9–11 years, and the last permanent teeth to erupt besides the wisdom teeth are the second permanent molars, at around 12–13 years of age.

7 *Correct answer D*: Only the premolars have two cusps (molars have at least four), but only the upper first premolar has two roots, arranged buccally and palatally. All other premolars have just one root.

8 *Correct answer C*: Upper canines usually have the longest roots of all the teeth, sometimes being longer than the usual endodontic file length of 25 mm, making root treatment of these teeth particularly difficult. Upper canines form the 'cornerstone' of the upper dental arch, giving the face structure and shape in this area. Their loss due to extraction leaves the face with a typical 'dished' appearance.

9 *Correct answer B*: Quadrant 4 in the FDI system is the lower right of the permanent dentition, and tooth 3 is the canine, so 43 is the lower right permanent canine tooth. The lower left first premolar will be charted as 34, the upper left first premolar will be charted as 24, and the upper right permanent canine will be charted as 13.

10 *Correct answer A*: The primary dentition does not have premolars and only two molar teeth, so the first molar is the only tooth that appears in both dentitions.

11 *Correct answer A*: This is the correct term to describe the natural shedding of the deciduous teeth as the permanent teeth begin to emerge, and it normally occurs between the ages of 6 years and 12 years – this is known as the mixed dentition stage. The abnormal loss of a tooth, usually carried out as a simple surgical procedure, is called extraction. Remineralisation is the process of enamel repair that occurs after demineralisation by the action of acids, and resorption is the natural loss of alveolar bone that occurs after a tooth has been extracted.

12 *Correct answer A*: The lower central incisors are narrower than the lateral incisors, and both lower teeth are smaller than the upper lateral incisors (unless these teeth develop abnormally as 'peg laterals'). The upper central incisor is the largest of the incisor teeth.

13 *Correct answer D*: The pulp is composed of soft tissue only, consisting of nerve fibres and blood vessels to form a neurovascular bundle within the pulp chamber of each tooth. All three of the other options are tooth tissues made up of calcium hydroxyapatite crystals in varying amounts.

14 *Correct answer C*: Although the deciduous teeth are smaller than their permanent successors, their pulp chambers are relatively larger and more likely to be breached at an early stage by caries. Deciduous teeth are lighter in colour and have the same number of cusps as their permanent successors, and the molars have characteristically divergent roots (curved outwards) to accommodate the crowns of the developing premolar teeth beneath them.

15 *Correct answer C*: The amelodentinal junction forms the inner base of both the enamel and dentine layers and is the point at which a carious attack becomes painful to the patient and requires restoration with a filling.

16 *Correct answer B*: The distal surface is the 'back' of a tooth and the most difficult to access when providing dental treatment to a tooth. The buccal surface is that adjacent to the cheeks and applies to all molars and premolars, the labial surface is that adjacent to the lips and applies to all the canines and

incisors, and the mesial surface is the 'front' of any tooth – that surface that lies closest to the midline of the dental arch.

17 *Correct answer C*: This ion exchange process produces a harder enamel surface that is more resistant to acid attack and is the basis for the use of fluoride-containing oral health products as well as topical and systemic fluoride applications.

18 *Correct answer C*: This term applies to all teeth in the lower arch, while the same surface in the upper arch teeth is referred to as palatal. The buccal surface is that adjacent to the cheeks and applies to all molars and premolars, and the labial surface is that adjacent to the lips and applies to all the canines and incisors.

19 *Correct answer C*: The oblique fibres form the majority of the fibres holding the tooth within the socket and run the full length of all the roots of each tooth. The alveolar crest fibres run from the bone crest to the neck of the tooth, while the apical fibres lie at the root apex only. Transeptal fibres run between the cementum of the adjacent teeth through the interdental regions.

20 *Correct answer A*: Cementum normally covers the dentine that makes up the inner structure of each root, whereas that dentine forming the crown of the tooth is covered with enamel. To hold the tooth in its socket, the periodontal ligament fibres engage anatomically with the cementum. This connection is destroyed when the tooth develops periodontal disease, and it gradually loosens as the underlying bone is also destroyed.

21 *Correct answer C*: This is the anatomical junction between the neck of the tooth and the gingival crevice soft tissue and is a specialised epithelial soft tissue that occurs nowhere else in the body. The attached gingiva is that which covers the majority of the alveolar process of bone, and the dentinocemental junction is the point within the tooth root where the cementum and root dentine are in contact with each other. The marginal gingiva forms the contoured gingival margins of the teeth.

22 *Correct answer B*: The junctional attachment is the point at which the epithelium of the gingiva physically attaches to the mineralised tissue of the tooth and normally lies at the deepest point of the gingival crevice. When a tooth has periodontal disease, the attachment remains but moves further down the length of the root as the disease progresses, so that a pocket is formed. It is the point that is probed during a periodontal examination to give a depth reading of the crevice or of a periodontal pocket if one is present. Food and drinks taken into the oral cavity for ingestion cannot pass beyond this point into the deeper periodontal tissues.

23 *Correct answer A*: As the gingivae swell up, they create the effect of the gingival crevice being deeper than its usual healthy depth of less than 3 mm. This gives the perceived effect of a periodontal pocket being present when it is not – hence the term false pocket. When the swelling and inflammation are resolved following oral hygiene measures, the gingival crevice returns to its usual appearance and depth.

24 *Correct answer B*: The free gingival fibres run from the cementum at the neck of the tooth into the soft tissue of the gingival papillae, and their elasticity maintains tension in the gingival tissues so that a tight cuff of tissue is present around the neck of each tooth.

25 *Correct answer C*: The minerals found in saliva include calcium and phosphates, and they act to buffer and stabilise the pH of the oral cavity, raising it from the critical pH 5.5 at which demineralisation of enamel occurs up to pH 7 (neutral). The bulk of saliva is composed of water that acts to carry the other constituents around the oral cavity. Antibodies and leucocytes (white blood cells) are present as part of the body's defence system against pathogens and disease.

26 *Correct answer B*: Mumps can affect one or both of the parotid glands, but does not affect any other. It is a viral infection caused by paramyxovirus, which usually occurs in childhood, although vaccination is available with the measles, mumps and rubella (MMR) vaccine.

27 *Correct answer D*: Salivary amylase (also known as ptyalin) is a digestive enzyme that acts on starch to begin carbohydrate digestion and is only found in saliva. Antibacterial enzymes are part of the defence mechanism and act against bacteria entering the mouth to prevent disease from occurring. Calcium phosphate is one of the minerals present that help to neutralise dietary acids and the weak organic acids formed by plaque bacteria, and immunoglobulin A is the most prevalent of the antibodies found in saliva as part of the immune system.

28 *Correct answer B*: Xerostomia is the condition of having a dry mouth and is due to age-related changes of the salivary glands or diseases such as Sjögren's syndrome. It can also occur as a side effect of various prescribed medications. All three of the other options may be seen in patients suffering from xerostomia, as the lubrication and cleansing effects of saliva are lost. The condition of having excessive salivation is called ptyalism.

29 *Correct answer C*: The head of the condyle is the ball-headed upper projection of the mandible that lies in the glenoid fossa of the temporal bone of the skull to form the temporomandibular joint. The joint is a hinged ball and socket type that allows the condylar head to glide, rotate and move laterally within the joint capsule.

30 *Correct answer A*: The lateral pterygoids are one of the four pairs of muscles of mastication that act to close the jaws and produce chewing movements. They are unique in that they can contract independently of one another, as well as together. They run between the lateral pterygoid plates of the skull and the condylar head of the mandible, with some fibres attaching to the cartilage meniscus of the joint itself. When both contract together, the mandible is pulled forwards so that the teeth can bite tip to tip.

31 *Correct answer D*: The motor component of the mandibular division of the trigeminal nerve supplies the muscles of mastication. The motor component of the facial nerve supplies the muscles of facial expression, and that of the glossopharyngeal nerve supplies the muscles of the pharynx, and the hypoglossal nerve supplies the muscles of the front of the tongue.

32 *Correct answer B*: The external carotid artery supplies oxygenated blood to the whole head outside of the cranium, including the oral cavity. The brain and other structures within the cranium are supplied by the internal carotid artery. All three of the other options supply oxygenated blood to their specific anatomical regions, and all are smaller branches off the carotid artery itself.

33 *Correct answer B*: The masseter muscles run from the outer surface of the zygomatic arch (the cheekbone) to the outer surface of the ramus and angle of the mandible on either side of the face, and when contracted, they are clearly visible in these areas as a knot of muscle. The temporalis muscle is visible in the temple region of the skull when it is clenched, but the two pterygoid muscles lie deep to the mandible and their contractions are not visible.

34 *Correct answer B*: All three of these nerves must be anaesthetised to ensure that both the tooth and its whole surrounding gingivae will not feel pain during the extraction procedure. The mental nerve is the end section of the inferior dental nerve and supplies all the teeth except the molars.

35 *Correct answer B*: The parotid glands are the only salivary glands to be innervated by the glossopharyngeal nerve, and several benign and malignant tumours are associated with them. The submandibular glands are innervated by the facial nerve and are most likely to be associated with salivary calculi (stones). The sublingual glands are also innervated by the facial nerve, while the accessory glands occur throughout the oral cavity and have various innervations depending on their location.

36 *Correct answer D*: The mental foramen lies on the outside surface of the mandible at a point between the roots of the lower premolar teeth, and the end section of the inferior dental nerve passes out of the mandible through it and onto the outer surface of the mandible. The incisive and lesser palatine foramina are features of the palatal part of the maxilla, and the infra-orbital foramen is a feature of the facial portion of the maxilla.

37 *Correct answer D*: This painful condition is an involuntary painful contraction of the muscles around the temporomandibular joint that prevents the mouth from being opened. It is often seen in patients who habitually clench and grind their teeth throughout the day and/or night, so that the muscles become overused, tired and then go into spasm. This parafunctional grinding habit is called bruxism.

38 *Correct answer B*: Leukoplakias are white patches seen on the oral soft tissues that have unknown causes and that often undergo sinister cell change to become malignant lesions. Their presence is therefore considered to be pre-malignant. All three of the other options are false statements.

39 *Correct answer B*: Patients with this condition are treated with drugs called bis-phosphonates, which are used to slow down the bone loss of the disease but which are linked with the occurrence of osteonecrosis. Those receiving the drugs by intravenous injections rather than in tablet form are more at risk of this side effect. Care should be taken when extracting teeth in this group of patients. There is no link between osteonecrosis and the other three options.

40 *Correct answer C*: *Candida albicans* is the fungus associated with thrush (oral and genital), and this infection is often seen in patients wearing dentures where the level of denture hygiene is poor. In denture stomatitis, the infection lies as white plaques on the palate, beneath the denture, which can be wiped away to reveal a red and raw-looking surface on the roof of the mouth. Treatment is with antifungal agents and to improve denture hygiene to an acceptable level.

41 *Correct answer D*: This is the typical appearance of an ulcer, although those associated with squamous cell carcinoma are usually painless and fail to heal. A cyst is an abnormal fluid-filled sac within the surrounding tissues, Leukoplakia appears as a white patch of unknown origin, and tumours occur as an over-growth of tissue with varying appearances depending on the tissue involved.

42 *Correct answer D*: These are large and painful ulcers that affect some patients but not others, and upon healing, the ulcer leaves a scar on the oral mucosa. They are not considered to be premalignant, whereas all three of the other options are so and the patient should be referred for specialist investigations.

UNIT 314
Dental Radiography

OUTCOME 1

Know the Regulations and Hazards Associated with Ionising Radiation

Questions

1 Under which one of the following circumstances must a radiation protection supervisor (RPS) be appointed in the dental workplace?
   A All workplaces taking dental pantomographs (DPT)
   B All workplaces using ionising radiation
   C All workplaces with a cephalostat machine
   D All workplaces with two or more x-ray machines

2 Which one of the following group of documents does not have to be stored in the radiation protection file?
   A Formal appointments
   B Local rules
   C Quality assurance programmes
   D Radiation qualification certificates

3 What is the correct term used to describe the 2 m distance around the x-ray machine head during exposures?
   A Contingency plan
   B Controlled area
   C Dose investigation level
   D Safety zone

4 In the event of an x-ray machine malfunction, the local rules will indicate the position of the machine isolator switch that will disconnect the electricity supply. Where should this information be displayed?
   A By the electricity fuse box
   B By the safety zone limit

Questions and Answers for Diploma in Dental Nursing, Level 3, First Edition. Carole Hollins.
© 2016 John Wiley & Sons, Ltd. Published 2016 by John Wiley & Sons, Ltd.

C By the x-ray control panel

D By the x-ray machine head

5 Radiation monitoring badges must be worn by the dental staff when a set number of intra-oral and/or extra-oral radiographs are exceeded in a week. What are the set numbers above which these monitoring devices must be in use?

A 10 extra-oral exposures

B 100 intra-oral exposures

C 150 intra-oral exposures

D 40 extra-oral exposures

6 Which of the following options represents the ionising radiation regulations concerned with the safety of patients while in the dental workplace?

A IR(ME)R 2000

B IRR99

C Local rules

D Radiation protection file

7 What is the title of the designated person appointed in each dental workplace to assess the risk of using ionising radiation and to oversee the precautions taken to minimise the risks identified?

A Legal person

B Medical physicist

C Radiation protection advisor

D Radiation protection supervisor

8 A designated controlled area must be identified around each x-ray machine in the dental workplace, as a circular area of 1.5 m around the machine. Which is the point from which this distance is measured?

A Dental chair

B Exposure button

C Machine control panel

D Machine head

9 Under IR(ME)R, the dose of radiation used should be in line with the ALARP (ALARA) principles at all times, so as low a dose as possible to produce a viable image should always be the goal to achieve. What is the correct term for this concept?

A Justification

B Optimisation

C Quality assurance

D Risk assessment

10 When is it acceptable for the x-ray machine to be switched on in the dental workplace?

A Before an exposure

B Each morning

C Start of each session

D Start of the week

11 The safe use of ionising radiation involves following the principle of ALARP (ALARA) to reduce the exposure of patients and staff to x-rays. Which one of the following will NOT help to achieve ALARP (ALARA)?

A Equipment maintenance

B Expose the patient only

C Fresh processing solutions

D Use of D-speed films

12 When an x-ray machine is in use, the beam of ionising radiation may scatter into the surrounding area. Which one of the following options assists in restricting the area of the beam, thereby reducing scatter?

A Collimator

B Fast film

C Intensifying screen

D Lead apron

13 Which one of the following actions cannot be carried out by an unqualified dental nurse?

A Change processing solutions

B Set exposure

C Process films

D Run a quality assurance audit

14 Which of the following options represents the ionising radiation regulations concerned with the safety of dental personnel while in the dental workplace?

A IR(ME)R 2000

B IRR99

C Local rules

D Radiation protection file

15 When tooth tissues are exposed to an x-ray beam, they absorb the rays at varying levels, depending on their mineral content. Which of the following terms describes those tissues that absorb little of the beam?

A Fluorescent

B Radiolucent

C Radiopaque

D Translucent

16 Which one of the following roles can be carried out by all dental staff, including the dental nurse?

   A IRMER practitioner

   B Operator

   C Radiation protection advisor

   D Referrer

17 Written information about the controlled area must be kept on the display at each x-ray machine in the dental workplace. How should this written information be referred to by dental personnel?

   A IR(ME)R 2000

   B IRR99

   C Local rules

   D Quality assurance programme

18 Under IR(ME)R, the benefit of exposing the patient to ionising radiation should be seen to outweigh the risk of causing tissue damage before an x-ray is taken. What is the correct term for this concept?

   A Justification

   B Optimisation

   C Quality assurance

   D Risk assessment

19 All dental workplaces using ionising radiation must undergo a 3-yearly assessment of radiation safety on the premises. Which one of the following organisations is most likely to undertake this assessment?

   A Care Quality Commission

   B Environmental Agency

   C Health and Safety Executive

   D Health Protection Agency

20 Where on the body is the recommended position to place a radiation monitoring badge, which is used to identify if a staff member has received any accidental exposures?

   A Chest area

   B Shoulder nearest the x-ray machine

   C Waist area

   D Wrist nearest the x-ray machine

Answers

1 *Correct answer B*: If ionising radiation is in use within the dental workplace, an RPS must be appointed as a legal requirement, irrespective of the number of machines or type of radiographs involved.

2 *Correct answer D*: The radiation protection file acts as a summary document that holds as much information as possible about the procedures in place to ensure radiation protection within the dental workplace. It must contain the details of all formal appointments (the names of all referrers, operators and so on, among the staff), the copies of the local rules for each x-ray unit on the premises and the details of all quality assurance programmes and audits that have been carried out. Qualification certificates for certain staff will be held in their personnel files, with a reference to them in the radiation protection file.

3 *Correct answer D*: The 2 m safety zone ensures that everyone is in a safe distance from the x-ray machine head and that only the patient remains within the 1.5 m controlled area during exposure. The additional half metre distance between the two measured areas is sufficient to prevent the staff members from being accidentally exposed to x-rays during their normal working day.

4 *Correct answer B*: The isolator switch must be positioned outside the controlled area so that it can be accessed safely without the risk of x-ray exposure to anyone who may need to use it in the event of an emergency but as close as safely possible to the x-ray machine so that it can be deactivated quickly to minimise the patient's x-ray exposure. The x-ray control panel and machine head will be within the controlled area, and the electricity fuse box could be anywhere on the premises and therefore is likely to be a long way from the scene of the emergency.

5 *Correct answer C*: A limit of 150 intra-oral exposures or 50 extra-oral exposures has been set, beyond which all staff members are legally required to wear a personal monitoring badge. These are worn at hip level and are sent for analysis to determine if they have been exposed to ionising radiation, usually once every 3 months. If the x-ray machines are being used correctly and are in a full working order and personnel are complying with IRR99, the monitoring badges should not register any exposure beyond the normal background levels. If exposure is detected, the cause can be investigated and rectified.

6 *Correct answer A*: These regulations are specifically concerned with the safety of patients who are exposed to ionising radiation during the production of medical images. IRR99 are specifically concerned with the safety of personnel working in premises where ionising radiation techniques are in use. Local rules show information that must be displayed for each x-ray machine under IRR99, and the radiation protection file is a summary document holding all of the relevant information under both IRR99 and IR(ME)R 2000, which must be maintained by the RPS.

7 *Correct answer D*: The radiation protection supervisor is a designated person within the workplace who may be a dentist or a dental care professional with a post-registration qualification in dental radiography. The legal person is usually the employer and their role is to ensure that the workplace complies fully with all ionising radiation regulations. The medical physicist is a specialist in ionising radiation and will be appointed as the radiation protection advisor for several dental workplaces.

8 *Correct answer D*: The source of the ionising radiation is held within the machine head, and the beam is emitted during exposure from this point, so the controlled area must be measured from here. The machine control panel will be in the controlled area but may be some distance from the radiation source, while the exposure button is portable and will be held outside the safety zone by the operator – at least 2 m from the source. The dental chair will be around 6 ft long and the x-ray head can be positioned at any point along it.

9 *Correct answer B*: Optimisation is to ensure that the lowest dose of ionising radiation possible is used for the shortest time and aimed at the smallest area of tissue possible to produce an image that is diagnostically acceptable. This will involve the use of fast films or intensifying screens, well-maintained machines that are fully functional, the skill of the operator to position the film and the patient correctly so that retakes are not necessary and so on, in line with ALARP/A.

10 *Correct answer A*: The machine takes a second to switch on and will function immediately, so there is no requirement for it to be left switched on at other times. To do so may also risk the staff and patients if the machine develops a fault and begins to leak radiation; this scenario would not come to light unless the staff happen to be wearing personal monitoring badges that would detect the unexpected radiation exposure when analysed – by which time the staff will have been irradiated for 3 months. Alternatively, a leak would not be discovered until the machine undergoes its three-yearly certification programme, by which time the staff may have received a dose sufficient to cause cell damage.

11 *Correct answer D*: Faster films are available for use (E speed and F speed), so the use of the slower D-speed films will increase radiation exposure, not decrease it in accordance with ALARP/A. A well-maintained equipment ensures their correct working and reduces the risk of accidental exposure, and the use of fresh processing solutions will have the same effect. Only the patient should be in the controlled area during an exposure.

12 *Correct answer A*: The rectangular collimator produces a parallel beam of radiation at the size of an intra-oral film, rather than the 'spray gun' effect of the old cone-type machines, so it reduces the scatter effect during the exposure. The use of fast films and intensifying screens helps to reduce the patient exposure, but they do not prevent scatter. Lead aprons are no longer recommended for use as an incorrect beam angulation may allow radiation beneath the apron so that both scatter and patient exposure will be increased, as the x-rays repeatedly bounce off the lead and re-expose the patient.

13 *Correct answer B*: Only a qualified dental nurse holding a dental radiography qualification can carry out this action, as it requires the knowledge and an understanding of the physics involved in the safe use of ionising radiation to be carried out correctly. Following suitable training, an unqualified (in training) dental nurse can carry out all three of the other duties listed.

14 *Correct answer B*: These regulations are specifically concerned with the safety of personnel working in premises where ionising radiation techniques are in use. IR(ME)R 2000 are concerned with the safety of patients who are exposed to ionising radiation during the production of medical images. The local rules are required to be displayed at each x-ray machine under IRR99, and the radiation protection file is a summary document holding all of the relevant information under both IRR99 and IR(ME)R 2000 for the safe use of ionising radiation on the premises.

15 *Correct answer B*: Radiolucent tissues tend to be hollow or soft tissues with little mineral content and therefore appear dark on the radiograph – such as a cavity in a tooth or a periapical abscess. Tissues and items with a high mineral content appear as grey/white features and are termed radiopaque – examples of these harder tissues include the bone and tooth enamel or items such as metal instruments. Fluorescent items are those where a chemical is exposed to radiation or electricity so that it glows from within – such as the rare earth chemicals used on intensifying screens. Translucent items are those that absorb little visible light and therefore appear 'see through'.

16 *Correct answer B*: Formal appointments are set out under IR(ME)R 2000, and the only appointment that is able to be held by a dental nurse is that of an operator. Only a dentist or specialist dental radiographer can be the referrer (the person who requests the exposure) or the IRMER practitioner (the person who justifies the exposure, by determining that the benefits to be gained will outweigh the radiation risk to the patient). The radiation protection advisor can only be a medical physicist and is appointed by the dental workplace as their source of specialist advice on matters relating to ionising radiation.

17 *Correct answer C*: Local rules are sets of information that are individual to each x-ray machine, and they must be displayed outside each room where an x-ray machine is present, under IRR99. The information they must contain includes the names of the RPS and the RPA, the designated controlled area for that particular machine and the contingency plan to be followed in the event of a malfunction of that particular machine.

18 *Correct answer A*: Each ionising radiation exposure must be justified by the IRMER practitioner – the benefits to be gained by the diagnosis of a problem must outweigh the risks to the patient of undergoing the exposure to be able to make that diagnosis. So the taking of 'routine' exposures, where nothing abnormal is expected to be seen, is not justified and should not be carried out. Optimisation is to ensure that the exposure is carried out in accordance with ALARP/A principles – the minimum radiation dose, for the shortest time and to the smallest area of body tissue to enable a diagnosis to be made.

19 *Correct answer D*: The Radiation Division of the Health Protection Agency (HPA) is the competent authority charged with the inspection and certification procedures that must be carried out on all ionising radiation machines, including those in the dental workplace. They have replaced the previous authority, the National Radiological Protection Board (NRPB). The HPA may send an engineer to attend in person to carry out the assessments, or they may issue the necessary test kits to the workplace with instructions on their use, and these are submitted for analysis by the HPA. If a problem with a machine is suspected, an engineer will then attend for further tests and investigations to be carried out.

20 *Correct answer C*: The most vulnerable area of the body to damage by exposure to ionising radiation is the reproductive organs, as there is a high cell turnover in these tissues, and they are therefore more at risk of undergoing cell change and mutation if they are hit during an exposure. The monitoring badge should therefore be worn at the waist level.

OUTCOME 2

Know the Different Radiographic Films and Their Uses

Questions

1 Horizontal bitewing radiographs are particularly useful views when diagnosing which one of the following conditions?
   A Interproximal caries of posterior teeth
   B Periapical abscess of a posterior tooth
   C Periodontal bone loss of posterior teeth
   D Unerupted canine

2 A dental pantomograph is one example of an extra-oral radiograph view. Which one of the following features of using this radiographic technique ensures that the x-ray exposure of the patient is kept to a minimum?
   A Fast films
   B Intensifying screens
   C Larger films
   D Light-tight cassette cases

3 Which one of the following options describes the correct angulation of the film that is necessary to be produced during the exposure of intra-oral film packets using a film holder?
   A Parallel to the tooth
   B Parallel to the x-ray beam
   C Perpendicular to the tooth
   D Perpendicular to the x-ray beam

4 Which one of the following options best describes the appearance of an acute periapical abscess on a radiograph?
   A Black area along the root
   B Rounded black area at the apex

Questions and Answers for Diploma in Dental Nursing, Level 3, First Edition. Carole Hollins.
© 2016 John Wiley & Sons, Ltd. Published 2016 by John Wiley & Sons, Ltd.

C White area along the root

D White-rimmed black area at the apex

5 When x-rays are directed at body tissues, the beam is absorbed at varying levels, depending on the mineral content of the tissue. Which one of the following terms describes those tissues that absorb little of the beam?

A Fluorescent

B Radiolucent

C Radiopaque

D Translucent

6 Which one of the following options correctly states the order of contents of an intra-oral film packet, from the x-ray machine tube side?

A Paper, film, foil, paper

B Paper, film, paper, foil

C Paper, foil, film, paper

D Paper, foil, paper, film

7 There are various intra-oral radiograph views available to the dental team. Which one of the following views will show the full length of one or two teeth and their surrounding bone?

A Anterior occlusal

B Horizontal bitewing

C Periapical

D Vertical bitewing

8 Which one of the following extra-oral radiograph views is produced using a machine called a cephalostat?

A Dental pantomograph

B Lateral oblique

C Lateral skull

D Orthopantomograph

9 Which one of the following options correctly lists the contents of an extra-oral film cassette, from the x-ray machine tube side?

A Film, intensifying screens, marker

B Intensifying screen, film, marker, intensifying screen

C Marker, film, intensifying screens

D Marker, intensifying screen, film, intensifying screen

10 Which one of the following intra-oral radiograph views is particularly useful for showing the presence of occlusal caries in several teeth?

A Anterior occlusal

B Horizontal bitewing

C Periapical

D Vertical bitewing

11 When x-rays are directed at body tissues, the beam is absorbed at varying levels, depending on the mineral content of the tissue. Which one of the following terms describes those tissues that absorb most of the beam?

A Fluorescent

B Radiolucent

C Radiopaque

D Translucent

12 What is the function of the lead foil within the intra-oral x-ray film packet?

A Absorbs scatter

B Allows the packet to be bent

C Focuses the x-ray beam

D Intensifies the image

13 Which one of the following views is taken to screen orthodontic patients for the presence or absence of teeth?

A Bitewing

B Cephalogram

C Dental pantomograph

D Lateral oblique

14 Which one of the following options is the particular feature of the technique using extra-oral film cassettes that ensures that the x-ray exposure of the patient is kept to a minimum?

A Intensifying screens fluoresce

B Special processing chemicals

C Use of automatic processor

D Use of large films

15 A tooth can be viewed as a digital image rather than as a conventional image. Which one of the following is not required to produce a digital image?

A Film

B Holder

C Rectangular collimator

D Sensor plate

16 Which one of the following intra-oral radiograph views is particularly useful when trying to determine if a patient has congenitally absent lateral incisor teeth?

A Horizontal bitewing

B Occlusal

C Periapical

D Vertical bitewing

17 Which one of the following options correctly identifies an important difference of a digital image over a conventional image of the same tooth?
   A Image is alterable
   B Image is darker
   C Image is permanent
   D Image is smaller

18 What is the purpose of using an intra-oral film holder when taking a horizontal bitewing view of a patient's teeth?
   A Allows a lower exposure time
   B Allows bisecting angle calculation
   C Allows film to be held still by the patient
   D Allows horizontal and vertical tube alignment

19 Which one of the following options is one of the main advantages of using digital radiographic techniques rather than conventional radiographic techniques?
   A Less costly
   B Reduced radiation dose
   C Sensor is smaller than film
   D Use of safer chemicals

20 Which one of the following options describes the purpose of intensifying screens within the cassettes used during extra-oral x-ray exposures?
   A Focus the x-ray beam
   B Glow to expose the film
   C Reflect more x-rays onto the film
   D Stop x-rays passing into the cassette

Answers

1 *Correct answer A*: This potential diagnosis is the main purpose of taking the horizontal bitewing view. A periapical abscess of any tooth is best diagnosed using a periapical view; suitable holders are available for both anterior and posterior teeth. Periodontal bone loss of posterior teeth is more easily seen using a vertical orientation of the bitewing view rather than a horizontal one, and an unerupted canine is diagnosed using either a periapical view or an anterior occlusal view.

2 *Correct answer B*: The inside leaves of all extra-oral cassettes are lined with an intensifying screen. This is coated with certain chemicals that fluoresce when exposed to ionising radiation, and the fluorescent glow creates the latent image on the encased film. This allows a lower exposure dose to be used than if the radiation had to penetrate the cassette and then be powerful enough to create the latent image on the film as well. Fast films are used for intra-oral views to reduce the exposure dose. Larger films and light-tight cassettes have no effect on reducing the exposure dose to the patient.

3 *Correct answer A*: This is the correct position used during the paralleling technique where, as the name suggests, the film packet is held parallel to the tooth to be viewed. If placed parallel to the x-ray beam, then no exposure would occur as the packet would lie along the beam, as it would if placed at 90° to the tooth. If the film packet is placed perpendicular to the x-ray beam, the image would be distorted unless the tooth also happened to be perpendicular to the beam too.

4 *Correct answer B*: This is the classic appearance of a periapical abscess, as a radiolucent circular ball of infection around the root apex. A black area along the root describes the typical appearance of a lateral periodontal abscess, while a corresponding white area indicates an area of increased mineralisation. A white-rimmed black area at the apex indicates a slow-growing lesion that is contained by the surrounding bone, such as a cyst, a tumour or a chronic infection.

5 *Correct answer B*: Radiolucent tissues tend to be hollow or soft tissues with little mineral content and therefore appear dark on the radiograph – such as a cavity in a tooth or a periapical abscess. Tissues and items with a high mineral content appear as grey/white features and are termed radiopaque – examples of these harder tissues include bone and tooth enamel, or items such as metal instruments. Fluorescent items are those where a chemical is exposed to radiation or electricity so that it glows from within – such as the rare earth chemicals used on intensifying screens. Translucent items are those that absorb little visible light and therefore appear 'see through'.

6 *Correct answer B*: The paper surrounds the film to protect it, and the foil behind the film absorbs any scatter of radiation. If the foil lies before the film, the majority of the radiation would be absorbed and very little (if any) radiation would penetrate and expose the film. The resultant image would not be of diagnostic value. If the foil and film lay against each other, it is likely that the film surface would be scratched and the image would be poor.

7 *Correct answer C*: This is the appearance of a typical periapical view, taken to show one or two teeth to their full length and including the surrounding bone and periodontal ligament area. An anterior occlusal view shows six or more teeth in full length, usually with some overlapping in the canine regions. Bitewing views will not show a tooth in full length.

8 *Correct answer C*: This is a specialist view that is often taken in complicated orthodontic cases, where the relationship of the jaws to the skull and to each other must be measured, assessed and monitored to determine the likely treatment plan to be followed. The cephalostat enables the patient's head to be held exactly in profile so that a true lateral image is produced, and the necessary measurements and angles can then be taken and calculated accordingly.

9 *Correct answer D*: The marker is present to indicate the patient's left side (usually) so that the view can be orientated correctly, and it must be superimposed onto the film during exposure. The film then lies between the pair of intensifying screens so that their fluorescence during exposure enables the latent image to be produced.

10 *Correct answer B*: All the views can be positioned to show several teeth, but the horizontal bitewing in particular will show the crowns of up to four teeth in both arches at a time, so eight teeth in total. Any or all of these teeth could be diagnosed with occlusal caries from just this one view. The vertical bitewing and the periapical views will show far fewer teeth, and the anterior occlusal view cannot be used to diagnose occlusal caries, as it cannot be positioned for posterior teeth.

11 *Correct answer C*: Tissues and items with a high mineral content will absorb much of the x-ray beam and will appear on film as grey/white features that are termed radiopaque – examples of these harder tissues include bone and tooth enamel, or items such as metal instruments like endodontic files, or metal pins and posts used during tooth restoration.

12 *Correct answer A*: Lead is a dense metal that prevents the passage of x-rays through its structure; rather, it absorbs the beam and therefore prevents scatter of any radiation that has passed through the anatomical structures under

exposure. The film packet should not be bent during use, as this will distort the image. An electrical current running across the beam is required to focus it, while special chemicals that fluoresce when exposed to radiation are required to intensify the image.

13 *Correct answer C*: This extra-oral view shows both upper and lower jaws, their surrounding bony anatomy and all of the teeth in two dimensions, with the presence or absence of any teeth quite being obvious to the viewer. The cephalogram is the lateral skull view that is taken for specific orthodontic cases only, while the lateral oblique view is used to locate the third molar teeth before extraction. The bitewing view is mainly taken for the detection of caries and is of no use for orthodontic screening purposes.

14 *Correct answer A*: The chemical coating on the screens will fluoresce when exposed to x-rays, and the high intensity of the resultant glow produces the latent image on the film. The same processing chemicals and automatic processor may be used for any type of intra- or extra-oral film, and larger films are required simply to record the full image.

15 *Correct answer A*: The sensor plate acts as the film with digital imagery techniques, and it passes the image produced directly to a computer screen, rather than requiring chemical processing once exposed. The rectangular collimator is still required to reduce scatter of the beam, and holders are used to align the sensor plate correctly, just as they do for film packets.

16 *Correct answer B*: The anterior occlusal view shows the full length of all four incisors and the canines, and the surrounding bone. The absence of the lateral incisor teeth will be obvious. Separate periapical views would have to be taken of both the left and right side to determine the presence or absence of the same teeth. Bitewing views are taken of posterior teeth.

17 *Correct answer A*: Computer software systems allow the digital image to be enhanced and altered on the screen, just as a digital photograph can. A conventional image is fixed onto the celluloid film and cannot be altered. The digital image will not be smaller or darker unless it has been deliberately altered using the computer software. Both images are permanent.

18 *Correct answer D*: The arm and ring extensions of the holder allow the tube to be correctly aligned both horizontally and vertically in relation to the film packet and the teeth. A bisecting angle technique is not used to produce the required image, and the use of a holder has no effect on the exposure time. Some patients may still tremble and wobble their jaw while biting onto the bite plate of the holder; its use does not prevent this from happening.

19 *Correct answer B*: The use of a sensor plate rather than a conventional film enables a lower dose of radiation to be used to create the required image. The sensor plate may be smaller than a conventional film, but this is not an advantage as fewer teeth may be viewed on each image and sometimes two images may be required to view all molars and premolars with horizontal bitewing views. Long teeth may not be also viewed in total with a digital technique. No chemicals are required to produce a digital image, so they are not safer than those used with conventional techniques.

20 *Correct answer B*: The screens fluoresce when exposed to ionising radiation, and the resultant glow produces the latent image on the film. This allows a lower exposure dose of radiation to be used to produce the image, which is safer for the patient and in line with the principles of ALARP/A. The x-ray beam can only be focused by an electrical current, while the screens do not act like a mirror to reflect the x-ray beam. If the x-ray beam cannot pass into the cassette, then the film cannot be exposed and the image will not be produced.

OUTCOME 3

Understand the Imaging Process and the Different Chemicals Used

Questions

1 Which one of the following events is prevented from happening during manual film processing, by replacing the lid of the developer tank after each use?
   A Contamination
   B Evaporation
   C Oxidation
   D Spillage

2 The dental terminology used to describe diagnostic items once they have been exposed and processed is quite distinct. Which one of the following terms correctly describes an item that is mounted on a viewer following processing?
   A Film
   B Film packet
   C Radiograph
   D X-ray film

3 Which one of the following options correctly lists the sequence of events to be carried out when manually processing a dental film?
   A Developer, fixer, wash
   B Developer, wash, fixer
   C Developer, wash, fixer, wash
   D Wash, developer, fixer, wash

Questions and Answers for Diploma in Dental Nursing, Level 3, First Edition. Carole Hollins.
© 2016 John Wiley & Sons, Ltd. Published 2016 by John Wiley & Sons, Ltd.

4 Which of the following statements is true with regard to the processing of radiographs?

   A Automatic processing is quicker than digital imaging

   B Automatic processors must be used under a safety light

   C Developer solution is alkaline

   D Fixer solution is classed as trade waste

5 Which one of the following states the light-sensitive chemicals that are used to coat the celluloid film within an intra-oral x-ray film packet?

   A Lead

   B Mercury

   C Rare earth chemicals

   D Silver bromide salts

6 What is the usual temperature range that is maintained during manual and automatic processing to ensure that the chemicals are at their most effective temperature of operation?

   A 15–17°C

   B 15–20°C

   C 18–22°C

   D 21–25°C

7 Which one of the following tasks must be carried out on a daily basis when manually processing radiographs but not when using an automatic processor?

   A Check solution temperatures

   B Provide water for wash tanks

   C Remove discarded film packets

   D Top up processing solutions

8 Various faults can occur on a radiograph during exposure to ionising radiation. Which one of the following options will produce a coned image?

   A Beam not central to film

   B Film placed backwards

   C Patient moved during exposure

   D Tube angle too shallow

9 A film has been loaded correctly into an automatic processing machine but does not appear in the delivery port at the end of the timed processing cycle. What is the most likely cause of this error?

   A Dirty rollers

   B Electrical fault

   C Inadequate levels of processing solutions

   D Low solution temperature

10 Various faults can occur during the processing of a film to produce a radiograph. Which one of the following options will produce a dark film?

A Developer solution too weak

B Developer solution too cold

C Incorrect processing sequence

D Over-developed

11 A periapical view of an upper central incisor tooth shows the tooth apex off the top of the film. What is the correct term for this fault?

A Coning

B Elongation

C Foreshortening

D Underexposure

12 While changing the automatic processing chemicals, a bottle is dropped and the fixer solution pours onto the bare arm of the dental nurse involved. Where will the potential first aid information regarding the fixer solution be located?

A COSHH file

B Infection control file

C Local rules

D Radiation protection file

13 The dental terminology used to describe diagnostic items is quite distinct. Which one of the following terms describes the item that is placed in the patient's mouth before exposure to ionising radiation?

A Film

B Film packet

C Radiograph

D X-ray film

14 Into which category of waste should spent developer and fixer solution be placed?

A Infectious hazardous waste

B Non-hazardous waste

C Non-infectious hazardous waste

D Trade waste

15 A set of bitewing radiographs have been processed, and the images produced appear indistinct and fogged. Which one of the following processing faults is most likely to have occurred?

A Developer solution too cold

B Exposed to light

C Fixer solution too hot

D Insufficient washing

16 Which light-sensitive chemicals are used to coat the celluloid film within an extra-oral x-ray film cassette?

A Lead

B Mercury

C Rare earth chemicals

D Silver bromide salts

17 Following an accidental spillage of fixer solution onto the floor, which one of the following solutions should be used to clean the area?

A Aldehyde solution

B Detergent solution

C Isopropyl alcohol solution

D Sodium hypochlorite solution

18 What is the correct term used to describe the process to be followed when an x-ray machine malfunctions, to ensure the safety of all persons present?

A Contingency plan

B Controlled area

C Local rules

D Risk assessment

19 A periapical view of a lower lateral incisor shows an image of the tooth that appears squashed and stunted, with no diagnostic value. Which one of the following exposure faults is likely to have caused this appearance?

A Coning

B Elongation

C Film movement

D Foreshortening

20 What is the recommended correct colour to be used for a safe light in the processing room, to avoid the unprocessed film becoming damaged by light exposure?

A Blue

B Red

C White

D Yellow

21 A periapical view has been taken of an upper incisor tooth, but while viewing the radiograph on the light box, the image appears to fade. Which one of the following processing faults is likely to have occurred?

A Developer solution too cold

B Developer solution too concentrated

C Inadequate fixing time

D Under-developed

22 An automatic processor will dry a processed radiograph before ejecting it from the machine at the delivery port. What is the likely appearance of a manually processed radiograph that has been dried too quickly by hand?

A Covered with crystalline debris

B Crazed pattern

C Scratched

D Stained green

23 What is the most likely result when a manually processed radiograph has been accidentally placed in the fixer solution before the developer solution?

A Blank film

B Dark film

C Faint image

D Fogged film

24 The automatic processor requires a draining, cleaning and replenishing routine carried out on a monthly basis to ensure its correct and optimal functioning. Which one of the following actions should be carried out first during this procedure?

A Drain the developer tank

B Drain the fixer tank

C Remove the rollers

D Switch the machine off

25 Which one of the following items of personal protective equipment is not suitable for use when draining, filling or topping up the automatic processor chemical tanks?

A Eye protection

B Gloves

C Plastic apron

D Visor

Answers

1 *Correct answer C*: The alkaline developer reacts with oxygen in the air so that its chemical composition is changed by oxidation, thereby destroying its ability to produce the latent image on the film. All of the tanks are able to be contaminated or spilled, while the developer solution is not volatile and will therefore not evaporate.

2 *Correct answer C*: The film packet contains the (x-ray) film that is exposed to ionising radiation to produce a latent (hidden) image. This is then chemically processed to become a radiograph that holds the permanent image.

3 *Correct answer C*: The film is inserted into the developer to enhance the latent image and then washed to remove any residual solution before being inserted into the fixer tank where the latent image becomes permanent. The films must be washed after each chemical immersion to remove residual chemicals and prevent contamination of the solutions.

4 *Correct answer C*: The alkaline developer solution reacts with the chemical coating of the film to produce the latent image, which is then made permanent by immersion into the acidic fixer solution, after washing. Both fixer and developer solutions are categorised as non-infectious hazardous waste, as they are potentially harmful to body tissues and require specialist disposal.

5 *Correct answer D*: The pungent smell of the used developer solution is bromine gas, and the slurry found in the base of the tank during cleaning is made up of silver salts. Rare earth chemicals are used in extra-oral cassettes to produce images with intensifying screens. Lead foil is found in intra-oral film packets to prevent radiation scatter, but mercury has no role in ionising radiation techniques.

6 *Correct answer C*: This maintains the processing chemicals at an average around that of room temperature, which is the optimum temperature required for the production of images on the films. All three of the other options are temperature ranges that are either too low or too high.

7 *Correct answer A*: The automatic processing machine controls the temperature of the solutions automatically, heating them if they are too low and maintaining them at room temperature otherwise. All three of the other options must be carried out daily for both manual and automatic processing systems.

8 *Correct answer A*: Part of the rectangular shape of the collimator will be seen to one side of the film, with the image cut off at its edges. A faint, patterned image will be produced if the film has been placed backwards, while a blurred image will occur if the patient moves during exposure. A shallow tube angle will produce an elongated image.

9 *Correct answer A*: The film will stick to the dirty rollers and remain somewhere within the machine itself – it will have to be dismantled to find the film, and the image is likely to be lost. The processing machine requires dismantling, cleaning and refilling on a monthly basis.

10 *Correct answer D*: Too long a time in the developer solution allows overproduction of the latent image, with loss of contrast between the dark and light areas of the image so that the whole film appears dark. A weak or cold developer solution will have the opposite effect, with only a faint image produced, while a blank film will result if it is placed in the fixer before the developer, as the latent image will be destroyed.

11 *Correct answer B*: The image appears stretched and longer than it should be, due to a shallow collimator angle producing an elongated image. Too steep an angle will produce a coned image, which appears squashed and stubby.

12 *Correct answer A*: COSHH stands for Control of Substances Hazardous to Health and is concerned with the risk assessment and identification of the safety precautions required for the safe use of all chemicals in the dental workplace. The file will hold any first aid measures required for each chemical if an accident occurs. All three of the other options will not hold this information.

13 *Correct answer B*: The x-ray film packet contains the unexposed film, surrounded by black paper and with a lead foil present on one side, all enclosed in a light-tight plastic packet. The film becomes a radiograph when processing has occurred and a permanent image has been produced.

14 *Correct answer C*: The processing chemicals are hazardous to humans, wildlife and the environment and must be collected and safely disposed of by specialist waste contractors. They are not infectious as the chemicals do not come into contact with body fluids.

15 *Correct answer B*: The film packets were either punctured due to poor storage procedures or opened for processing in an area that was not light-tight. Visible light has fallen on the films and partially destroyed the latent images before they were fixed onto the radiographs.

16 *Correct answer C*: These chemicals react to the fluorescent glow produced by the intensifying screens on exposure to ionising radiation, creating the latent image on the film, which is then formed into a permanent image during processing. Silver bromide salts are the chemicals found on intra-oral films before processing.

17 *Correct answer B*: A general-purpose detergent cleaner will remove the spillage adequately, without releasing any noxious vapours that may occur with any of the other three options.

18 *Correct answer A*: The contingency plan will form part of the local rules that are displayed outside each room where ionising radiation is in use and will detail the safe actions to take in the event of a malfunction, so that all persons come to no harm. The local rules are a set of operational and safety instructions to be followed for each machine and must be displayed in accordance with IRR99.

19 *Correct answer D*: The angulation of the collimator was too steep, so that the x-ray beam has exposed the tooth at a severe angle. This produces a squashed and stunted appearance of the tooth, as the beam has passed almost down the long axis of the tooth, rather than at 90° to it as it should have done.

20 *Correct answer B*: The chemicals present on the film are most sensitive to light at the blue end of the electromagnetic spectrum, so the safest colour of the light will be at the opposite end, in the red zone. White light is visible light, and this does contain blue light too.

21 *Correct answer C*: The film must be immersed in the fixer solution for long enough that the image becomes permanent. If it is too short a time, the image will gradually fade as the film is viewed in visible light. A cold developer solution, or too short a time immersed in it, will result in a faint image, while too concentrated a solution will produce a black film as it has been over-developed.

22 *Correct answer B*: Various techniques are used to quickly dry a manually processed radiograph, from the use of a hair dryer to hanging it over a radiator. If dried too quickly over a strong heat source, the celluloid film itself becomes damaged and distorted and the overlying chemical film will crack and lie in a crazed pattern. If the film is inadequately fixed, it will have green stains present, whereas crystalline debris on the film indicates that insufficient washing has occurred. A scratched film has been mishandled during the processing procedure.

23 *Correct answer A*: The latent image will be destroyed as the silver bromide salts are stripped from the celluloid base, and the film will appear blank.

24 *Correct answer D*: Any electrically operated machinery must be disconnected from its power supply before being dismantled, whether for cleaning purposes or for repair. This is a basic safety measure to prevent injury or electrocution of staff members, especially with electrical machinery that uses fluids and water.

25 *Correct answer D*: A visor will not prevent the inhalation of fumes from the processing chemicals – a face mask must be worn instead. All three of the other items of PPE should also be worn when handling large volumes of these chemicals.

Understand the Importance for Stock Control of Radiographic Films

Questions

1 An anterior occlusal radiograph has been taken to determine the positions of both unerupted upper canine teeth. Which one of the following options should be used to determine the correct orientation of the radiograph, so that the left and right teeth can be separately identified?
   A Crowns to the top
   B Pimple forwards
   C Pimple in the upper left corner
   D Tooth roots to the top

2 When scoring during a quality assurance analysis of radiographs, some may be marked as having errors present that prevent a diagnosis being made. Which one of the following options does this statement describe?
   A Score 1
   B Score 2
   C Score 3
   D Score 4

3 Which one of the following options is true, with regard to the correct storage of X-ray film stock?
   A Fast films must be kept in their original package
   B Films do not have 'use by' dates, like chemicals
   C Old and new stock must not be stored together
   D Old stock must be used first

Questions and Answers for Diploma in Dental Nursing, Level 3, First Edition. Carole Hollins.
© 2016 John Wiley & Sons, Ltd. Published 2016 by John Wiley & Sons, Ltd.

4 Which of the following options is false with regard to the storage of digital images of the teeth?

A Can be emailed to colleagues

B Can be stored on a disc

C Cannot be allocated to another patient

D Cannot be printed out

5 When a periapical view of an upper incisor is mounted for viewing, which one of the following correctly describes the orientation of the film on the viewer?

A Incisor root above the crown

B Mesial edge of the tooth to the right of the film

C Pimple in the bottom left corner of the film

D Pimple in the top left corner of the film

6 The aim of a quality assurance programme of radiographs is to keep exposure and processing faults to a minimum. Which one of the following is the current ratio of acceptable ratings for processed films?

A Score 1, 10% minimum

B Score 1, 70% maximum

C Score 3, 10% maximum

D Score 3, 70% minimum

7 Which one of the following storage conditions will not affect the shelf life of X-ray film packets, by causing their deterioration before reaching the stated expiry date?

A Close source of ionising radiation

B Cold stock room

C Damp packaging

D Hot cupboard

8 When a dental pantomograph (DPT) is mounted for viewing by the dentist, which one of the following correctly describes the orientation of the film on the viewer?

A The left maxillary molars will be on the dentist's bottom left

B The left maxillary molars will be on the dentist's bottom right

C The left maxillary molars will be on the dentist's top left

D The left maxillary molars will be on the dentist's top right

9 A left horizontal bitewing radiograph has been taken to determine if the first molar teeth have occlusal caries present. The image is coned and the second molars have been missed off the exposure. What is the most likely quality assurance rating for this radiograph?

A Score 1

B Score 2

C Score 3

D Score 4

10 A periapical radiograph of the upper left first premolar tooth (24) shows distal caries present. However, the radiograph has been mounted back to front and then viewed several days later. What is the possible consequence of this error?
  A Distal restoration of 14
  B Distal restoration of 24
  C Mesial restoration of 14
  D Mesial restoration of 24

11 After processing, a radiograph appears black and no image is visible. What is the quality assurance rating of this film?
  A Score 1
  B Score 2
  C Score 3
  D Score 4

12 When run correctly, a quality assurance system of radiographs has to achieve which one of the following aims?
  A Be cost-effective
  B Minimise patient exposure to an acceptable level
  C Reduce patient waiting times
  D Save clinical time

13 Clinical governance guidelines set out the acceptable percentage scores of analysed radiographs as a maximum of poor quality and a minimum of excellent quality. Which one of the following options correctly states these scores?
  A Excellent minimum 10%, poor maximum 70%
  B Excellent minimum 30%, poor maximum 10%
  C Poor maximum 10%, excellent minimum 70%
  D Poor maximum 30%, excellent minimum 70%

14 Which one of the following options describes the correct system of film stock rotation in their designated storage area?
  A New stock at the back
  B Pimple facing backwards
  C Pimple facing forwards
  D Separate shelf for each film size

15 When scoring during a quality assurance analysis of radiographs, some may be marked as having minimal errors present that do not prevent a diagnosis being made. Which one of the following options does this statement describe?
  A Score 1
  B Score 2
  C Score 3
  D Score 4

16 Which one of the following statements is false in relation to the running of a quality assurance programme of radiographs in the dental workplace?
  A Identifies exposure faults
  B Identifies justified exposures
  C Identifies machine malfunction
  D Identifies processing faults

17 Which one of the following describes an unacceptable method of storage of X-ray film packets in the dental workplace?
  A Cupboard in stock room with filling materials
  B Cupboard next to X-ray machine
  C Drawer in processing room
  D Drawer in surgery with instruments

18 When a set of horizontal bitewing radiographs are correctly mounted for viewing, which one of the following descriptions will not be seen?
  A The dental arch will curve up on the outer sides of the radiographs
  B The molar teeth will be on the outer sides of the radiographs
  C Pimples will face outwards towards the person viewing
  D Root apices will be at the top and bottom of the radiographs

19 A periapical radiograph has been taken of the lower right second premolar tooth that is undergoing endodontic treatment and root filling, and the view has been coned so that just the crown of the tooth is missing from the radiograph. Which of the following is the most likely quality assurance rating for this view?
  A Score 1
  B Score 2
  C Score 3
  D Score 4

20 When scoring during a quality assurance analysis of radiographs, some may be marked as having no errors present. Which one of the following options does this statement describe?
  A Score 1
  B Score 2
  C Score 3
  D Score 4

Answers

1 *Correct answer B*: All intra-oral radiographs are first aligned by having the raised pimple of the film facing forwards – this correctly determines left from right. The radiograph is then turned up or down depending on whether the upper or lower teeth are to be viewed; for this scenario, the tooth roots will be at the top of the film as the upper teeth are being viewed. Orientating the film initially to have the roots at the top does not distinguish left from right, and it may then be viewed back to front.

2 *Correct answer C*: Score 3 is given when an exposure, handling or processing fault has rendered the radiograph unreadable, so that a diagnosis cannot be made from it and the view must be taken again. There is no score 4.

3 *Correct answer D*: The chemicals on the celluloid film within the packet will deteriorate over time so that the films become unusable – they do have 'use by' (expiry) dates. It is important therefore that stock is rotated and old films are used first to avoid waste. Stock is normally kept together in storage, with new products being placed behind old packets, and it is usual to keep the packet in storage and place a few films at a time in the clinical area for easy access.

4 *Correct answer D*: As with digital photographs, digital radiograph images can easily be printed onto ordinary paper from the computer hard drive. All three of the other options are true.

5 *Correct answer A*: Of the options given, this is the only correct orientation of the radiograph as it mimics the actual position of the tooth in the jaw bone. Having the mesial edge of the tooth to the right of the film is only correct when viewing the upper right incisors, and the pimple can be located in any corner of the radiograph as long as it faces forwards; its position is not used to orientate the radiograph.

6 *Correct answer C*: Score 3 indicates a film that is diagnostically unacceptable and will need to be retaken; the acceptable percentage of these per 100 radiographs is a maximum of 10%. Score 1 indicates an excellent quality radiograph with no faults, and the acceptable percentage of these is a minimum of 70% per 100 radiographs.

7 *Correct answer B*: Heat, damp and accidental exposure to ionising radiation will all affect stored film packets detrimentally. A cold stock room will not have this effect, as film packets can be stored safely down to 10°C.

8 *Correct answer D*: With the left maxillary molars on the dentist's top right, the radiograph is orientated the same as if the dentist is looking into the patient's mouth – this is the correct view. If these teeth are on the dentist's top left, the film is back to front, and if they are on the bottom, the film is upside down and back to front when on the bottom right.

9 *Correct answer B*: The radiograph has been taken to view the first molar teeth in particular. These are present on the view and a diagnosis can be made, but the coned image prevents a score 1, which is excellent quality with no faults. A score 2 is given as the image is diagnostically acceptable despite a fault being present. If the first molar teeth had been missed off the view, a score 3 would have been given as the image would have been diagnostically unacceptable and requiring a retake.

10 *Correct answer A*: With the film mounted back to front, the tooth will appear to be the upper right first premolar (14), although the caries will still be visible distally. A possible consequence will then be an unnecessary distal restoration of the upper right first premolar tooth.

11 *Correct answer C*: Score 3 indicates a diagnostically unacceptable image, which will require a retake. There is no score 4.

12 *Correct answer B*: The aim of the quality assurance system is to achieve ALARP/A – the principle of keeping all exposures of the patient to ionising radiation to a minimum or 'as low as reasonably possible' (practicable/acceptable). The quality assurance system should analyse the quality of the radiographs taken and determine the percentage that have faults, how the faults occurred and how to avoid them in the future. This will reduce the number of retakes and minimise patient exposure. All three of the other options have no bearing on the correct running of the system.

13 *Correct answer C*: Score 3 indicates poor quality and should be a maximum of 10% per 100 films analysed, while score 1 indicates excellent quality and should be a minimum of 70% per 100 films.

14 *Correct answer A*: Old film stock must be at the front on the storage shelf so that it is used first, before it passes its expiry date. New stock must therefore be placed behind it. Separate shelves are not necessary for different film sizes, and the position of the pimple is only relevant on a processed radiograph to ensure it has been orientated correctly for viewing purposes.

15 *Correct answer B*: Score 2 radiographs are of good enough quality to enable a diagnosis to be made but have a fault present. However, the fault does not prevent diagnosis. There is no score 4.

16 *Correct answer B*: The justification for carrying out the exposure is a decision made by the IRMER practitioner beforehand, by determining that the diagnostic benefits gained will outweigh the risks of the exposure to the patient. All exposures should therefore be justified. All three of the other options are true statements.

17 *Correct answer B*: When the X-ray machine is switched on before, during and after an exposure, it is possible for ionising radiation to leak from the radiation source unknowingly. If the unexposed film packets are stored close to this radiation source, it is possible that they will be inadvertently exposed and therefore will be useless for controlled exposures in the future. All film packets should be stored as far away from the X-ray machine as possible. All three of the other options are acceptable storage sites.

18 *Correct answer D*: Bitewing radiographs cannot be positioned to show root apices; periapical views are required for this. All three of the other options are correct when viewing correctly mounted bitewing radiographs.

19 *Correct answer B*: The justification for this exposure will be to determine the working length of the root canal or to indicate an adequate root filling to that working length. In both cases, the root apex must be shown on the radiograph, but the crown of the tooth is not vital. Score 2 indicates a diagnostically acceptable radiograph with a fault present that does not prevent that diagnosis. There is no score 4.

20 *Correct answer A*: Score 1 indicates an excellent quality radiograph with no exposure, handling or processing errors present – it is the best score to be aspired to and should make up no less than 70% of radiographs taken by an operator.

OUTCOME 1

Know the Common Oral Diseases

Questions

1 Which one of the following is the most likely presentation of an early carious area in a tooth?
   A Cavity
   B Periapical abscess
   C Reversible pulpitis
   D White spot lesion

2 Which one of the following terms is used to describe a disease condition involving the inflammation of the supporting structures of the tooth?
   A Apical abscess
   B Dental caries
   C Gingivitis
   D Periodontitis

3 The formation of a carious lesion in a previously sound tooth follows a set sequence. Which one of the following events describes the final stage of this sequence, of those options shown below?
   A Caries enters the dentine layer
   B Caries enters the enamel layer
   C Caries reaches the amelodentinal junction
   D Demineralisation of the enamel

4 Which one of the following microorganisms is not involved with the production of weak organic acids associated with enamel demineralisation?
   A *Lactobacillus*
   B *Staphylococcus aureus*
   C *Streptococcus mutans*
   D *Streptococcus sanguis*

Questions and Answers for Diploma in Dental Nursing, Level 3, First Edition. Carole Hollins.
© 2016 John Wiley & Sons, Ltd. Published 2016 by John Wiley & Sons, Ltd.

5 Bacterial plaque is linked with the development of both dental caries and periodontal disease. Which one of the following describes the role of plaque in caries formation rather than in periodontal disease?

A Acid formation

B Poor oral hygiene

C Presence of bacteria

D Presence of saliva

6 Which one of the following options is an example of a non-milk extrinsic sugar?

A Dextrose

B Fructose

C Lactose

D Maltose

7 Which one of the following is the term used to describe non-carious tooth tissue loss caused by bruxism?

A Abfraction

B Abrasion

C Attrition

D Erosion

8 Which one of the following factors is relevant to the development of gingivitis?

A Bacterial plaque

B Carbohydrate foods

C Frequency of acid attacks

D Weak organic acids

9 Periodontal disease can be exacerbated by many medical factors. Which one of the following conditions is not directly linked to a worsening severity of periodontal disease?

A Asthma

B Diabetes

C Stress

D Vitamin C deficiency

10 There are many different types of bacteria normally present in the oral cavity. Which one of the following organisms is usually associated with the onset of dental caries?

A *Actinomyces*

B *Bacteroides*

C *Lactobacillus*

D *Streptococcus*

11 Various microorganisms can infect the body to cause diseases. Which one of the following describes a microorganism in its non-infective state?

A Bacterium

B Fungus

C Spore

D Virus

12 Which one of the following options is the correct term used to describe the condition where a tooth experiences pain from a caries attack that can be resolved by removing the caries and filling the cavity?

A Cellulitis

B Glossitis

C Pericoronitis

D Pulpitis

13 The body has several lines of defence that should protect a person from a disease developing and making them ill. Which one of the following options listed is the last line of defence available before the disease process takes hold?

A Inflammatory response

B Mucous membrane

C Saliva

D Skin

14 Which one of the following terms correctly describes the second condition that a patient may experience when a tooth undergoes a carious attack?

A Acute alveolar abscess

B Chronic alveolar abscess

C Irreversible pulpitis

D Reversible pulpitis

15 Bacterial plaque is often described as a transparent biofilm. Which one of the following components of this biofilm is not always present in samples of plaque within the oral cavity?

A Food debris

B Microorganisms

C Oral debris

D Saliva

16 During an attack by pathogenic microorganisms, many defence cells and pathogens are killed and pus forms. Which one of the following terms describes the condition where pus spreads uncontrolled into the surrounding tissues?

A Abscess

B Acute infection

C Cellulitis

D Chronic infection

17 During the progression of periodontal disease, various anaerobic bacteria colonise the plaque as it extends subgingivally. Which one of the following is an example of one of these types of bacteria?

A *Actinomyces*

B *Lactobacillus*

C *Staphylococcus*

D *Streptococcus*

18 The formation of a carious lesion in a previously sound tooth follows a set sequence. Which one of the following events describes the first stage of this sequence, of those options shown below?

A Caries enters the dentine layer

B Caries enters the enamel layer

C Caries reaches the amelodentinal junction

D Demineralisation of the enamel

19 Which one of the following stagnation areas is associated with the development of periodontal disease?

A Buccal pit

B Denture clasp

C Gingival crevice

D Interproximal area

20 Many patients are diagnosed with the condition of chronic gingivitis. Which one of the following options listed is usually the first stage in the development of this condition?

A Development of false pockets

B Development of subgingival calculus

C Mineralisation of plaque

D Production of toxins

21 Which one of the following signs of inflammation is usually the last one to occur?

A Heat

B Loss of function

C Pain

D Swelling

22 Various medical conditions, or the drugs prescribed to treat them, may aggravate the severity of periodontal disease. Which one of the following options is a medical condition that is often linked to the presence of false pockets in the sufferer?

A Diabetes

B Epilepsy

C Leukaemia

D Vitamin C deficiency

23 Bacterial plaque is linked with the development of both dental caries and periodontal disease. Which one of the following describes the main role of plaque in the onset and progression of periodontal disease rather than in caries formation?

A Acid formation

B Poor oral hygiene

C Presence of bacteria

D Presence of saliva

24 The measure of acidity or alkalinity of a solution is called its pH level. Which one of the following is the pH level at which enamel demineralisation first begins?

A pH 2.5

B pH 5.5

C pH 7.5

D pH 9.5

25 Which one of the following options is a feature of chronic periodontitis but not of chronic gingivitis?

A Bleeding on probing

B Gingival inflammation

C Subgingival calculus

D True pocket

26 Which one of the following relevant factors in the development of dental caries can be most easily controlled by the patient to reduce their own caries experience and improve their oral health?

A Bacterial production of weak organic acids

B Consumption of carbohydrate in the diet

C Length of time and frequency of acid attacks

D Presence of certain bacteria in the oral cavity

27 Which one of the following microscopic cells is responsible for the production of secondary dentine following a carious attack on a tooth?

A Ameloblasts

B Cementoblasts

C Odontoblasts

D Osteoblasts

28 Established periodontal disease may be worsened by certain other aggravating factors. Which one of the following is an aggravating factor that may be prevented by the provision of dentures?

A Hormonal changes

B Mouth breathing

C Smoking

D Unbalanced occlusion

29 Which one of the following options is the correct term used to name a yellow-coloured, hard deposit that is often visible in the oral cavity of patients with a poor standard of oral hygiene?

A Biofilm

B Plaque

C Subgingival calculus

D Supragingival calculus

30 Which one of the following statements is false in relation to the development and progression of chronic periodontal disease?

A Anaerobic bacteria attack alveolar bone causing tooth mobility

B Micro-ulcers allow toxins into the soft tissues

C Subgingival calculus has an overlying layer of plaque present

D True pockets form as the periodontal ligament is destroyed

Answers

1 *Correct answer D*: A white spot lesion indicates an area of initial demineralisation of the enamel. An established lesion will present as a cavity, and the pulp will become inflamed as the caries extends deeper through the dentine, so the tooth develops reversible pulpitis. Once the pulp chamber has been breached and the tooth dies, a periapical abscess will develop on the end of the root.

2 *Correct answer D*: The supporting structures of the teeth are the gingivae, the periodontal ligament, the alveolar bone and the cementum, which lines the root dentine. Collectively, they are referred to as the periodontium, and when inflamed, they are said to have periodontitis.

3 *Correct answer A*: The sequence of events of the options shown is as follows: the enamel demineralises, the caries enters the enamel layer, the caries reaches the amelodentinal junction (the junction between the enamel and dentine), and then the caries enters the dentine layer.

4 *Correct answer B*: The microorganisms that produce weak organic acids that demineralises the enamel are those associated with dental caries. *Staphylococcus aureus* is a microorganism that does not usually occur in the oral cavity and is associated with skin boils and infections. All three of the other options are bacteria associated with the onset and progression of caries.

5 *Correct answer A*: The bacteria within the plaque produce weak organic acids as they digest carbohydrate-based food debris in the mouth, which then causes enamel demineralisation. This acid has no effect on the periodontal tissues. All three of the other options are relevant to bacterial plaque involved with caries and periodontal disease.

6 *Correct answer A*: Non-milk extrinsic sugars are those that are not present naturally in food products nor milk-based, but are added artificially by the food manufacturer. Dextrose is a non-milk extrinsic sugar that is a form of glucose and is artificially added to many food products. Fructose is an intrinsic sugar found in fruits, lactose is an extrinsic sugar found in milk, and maltose is an intrinsic sugar of starchy vegetables and grasses, such as sugar beet and sugar cane.

7 *Correct answer C*: Bruxism is the habitual act of clenching and grinding the teeth together, so that their occlusal surfaces and incisal edges become worn down. The non-carious tooth surface loss that results is called attrition. Abfraction is the specific sudden loss of a section of tooth from the cervical region and is due to shearing forces on the tooth. Abrasion is the gradual loss of tooth tissue from the buccal and labial surfaces due to heavy or vigorous toothbrushing. Erosion is the loss of tooth tissue due to the action of dietary acids on the enamel.

8 *Correct answer A*: Plaque bacteria lying in the gingival crevice or along the gum line release toxins that cause inflammation of the local gingivae, unless the plaque is removed by toothbrushing. All three of the other options are relevant to the onset of dental caries rather than gingivitis.

9 *Correct answer A*: There is no medical link between this respiratory condition and periodontal disease. However, all three of the other options are known risk factors in the progression of established periodontal disease, although they do not cause the disease itself. Diabetes in particular has a worsening effect on the condition, as the reduced peripheral blood flow associated with the condition causes poor wound healing generally for sufferers.

10 *Correct answer D*: *Streptococcus mutans* is the particular microorganism that first colonises plaque and produces the weak organic acids responsible for demineralisation and early carious lesions. Species of *Lactobacillus* are found in established carious cavities only, and the other two options are microorganisms associated with periodontal disease.

11 *Correct answer C*: This is the dormant state of bacteria, where they exist in a protective shell and are unreactive to their surroundings. They exist and survive in this state when exposed to a harsh environment, such as extremes of temperature or drought conditions.

12 *Correct answer D*: The inner core of a tooth is made up of a neurovascular bundle called the pulp, and this is the soft tissue that becomes inflamed during a caries attack. Its nerve endings lie in tubules within the dentine and are sensitised when the caries reaches this tooth layer. If the caries is removed at this point and the tooth restored, the pain goes. This is reversible pulpitis.

13 *Correct answer A:* The skin and mucous membranes provide a physical defence barrier to any potential pathogens, while saliva contains defence leucocytes that attack and destroy microorganisms that enter the mouth. If pathogens gain entry to the deeper tissue layers past these lines of defence, an inflammatory response develops to fight the microorganisms at a cellular level.

14 *Correct answer C*: The initial condition is reversible pulpitis as the caries reaches the dentine layer of the tooth. This becomes irreversible pulpitis when the pulp chamber is breached. The pulp will then die quickly and an acute apical abscess will form, or it will die slowly and a chronic apical abscess will form.

15 *Correct answer A*: Bacterial plaque is present in the mouth at all times – it does not develop only while food is being consumed. It always consists of microorganisms, saliva and oral debris (such as epithelial cells that constantly detach from the oral mucous membranes), but it will only contain food debris when food is consumed. So after bedtime toothbrushing, the plaque found on the teeth and soft tissues the following morning will not contain food debris.

16 *Correct answer C*: This is a spreading infection throughout several layers of the body tissues at the same time, which often requires intensive medical care to treat. The infection states associated with the other three options tend to be contained within a single tissue layer.

17 *Correct answer A*: Oxygen levels are reduced dramatically as periodontal pockets develop and plaque extends subgingivally. The bacteria found here are able to survive in these low-oxygen environments and are called anaerobic bacteria. *Actinomyces* is one such microorganism species, while all of the other three options are aerobic bacteria that live in high-oxygen environments.

18 *Correct answer D*: The surface of the enamel is first demineralised by the weak organic acids produced by the caries bacteria, and then the enamel is breached. The caries front continues through the enamel until it reaches the amelodentinal junction and then crosses into the deeper dentine layer of the tooth.

19 *Correct answer C*: Plaque that is allowed to accumulate in the gingival crevice due to poor toothbrushing techniques will cause gingivitis and eventually periodontitis as the supporting structures are damaged. All three of the other options are stagnation areas that are likely to result in the onset of caries, as the plaque lies against the tooth in each instance.

20 *Correct answer D*: The bacteria within plaque produce toxins that act to irritate the gingival tissues and cause them to swell. The gingival hyperplasia that results is associated with false pockets (pockets due to tissue swelling rather than tissue destruction). The plaque becomes mineralised by incorporating minerals from saliva, and this develops first above and then below the gingival margin as supragingival and then subgingival calculus.

21 *Correct answer B*: The heat and swelling that occur due to the sudden increased blood flow to the area cause the compression of nerve fibres in the immediate vicinity, and the area becomes painful. The discomfort that occurs due to these other signs will finally cause the patient to stop using the tissue affected; so pulp inflammation eventually stops the patient from chewing with the affected tooth.

22 *Correct answer B*: A common anti-epileptic drug is prescribed to prevent the occurrence of further fits once a patient has been diagnosed with epilepsy. Called phenytoin (Epanutin), it has the side effect of causing gingival

hyperplasia, often in the absence of plaque, and patients are plagued by the presence of false pockets. These create stagnation areas and make adequate plaque removal difficult, and sufferers may have to undergo gingival re-contouring on a regular basis.

23 *Correct answer B*: Plaque remaining in the gingival crevice or within existing pockets will cause gingivitis or exacerbate periodontitis. Consistently, poor oral hygiene levels will result in periodontal disease eventually, whereas the onset of caries depends more on the diet content and the frequency of consumption of non-milk extrinsic sugars and dietary acids. Patients who do not consume these types of foods and drinks tend not to develop caries, even when their oral hygiene is poor.

24 *Correct answer B*: This is also called the critical pH, the point at which the oral cavity is just acidic enough for enamel demineralisation to begin. If the pH is neutralised and raised towards 7, the demineralisation stops.

25 *Correct answer D*: True pockets are formed down the sides of the tooth roots as the supporting tissues are destroyed by the advancement of subgingival calculus and aerobic bacteria in the overlying plaque. Their presence is a diagnostic feature of chronic periodontitis.

26 *Correct answer C*: Many foods contain 'hidden sugars' that have been introduced by the manufacturers for a variety of reasons into foods that would not normally be associated with sugar. A classic example is tomato-based products such as soups and sauces – these are savoury products that should not (and do not) taste sweet, but contain a considerable amount of cariogenic additions. The patient has no control over their presence in these foods. However, they can control the number of times cariogenic foods and drinks are taken throughout the day and for how long a time their teeth are exposed to these products. The presence of bacteria in the mouth and their activity to produce acids are not controllable.

27 *Correct answer C*: Odontoblasts are the cells that lay down dentine, whether primary or secondary dentine. Ameloblasts lay down the enamel, cementoblasts lay down the cementum, and osteoblasts lay down the bone.

28 *Correct answer D*: Many patients have posterior teeth extracted and are left to nibble foods with their remaining anterior teeth. These developed to be used to bite into foods initially rather than to perform the chewing actions themselves, but they must perform this function in the absence of posterior teeth. This puts unnatural forces on the anterior teeth that, in the presence of periodontal disease, will become loose in their sockets and begin to move – often, the upper incisors in particular become severely proclined and spaced out. The provision of dentures to replace the missing teeth provides a more balanced occlusion and prevents the uneven forces on the remaining teeth.

29 *Correct answer D*: This is the typical appearance of supragingival calculus – that above the gum line and visible in the mouth. Subgingival calculus is dark brown or black and is not visible as it lies below the gum line. Plaque is a soft, white layer of debris on the teeth or gingival margins, and the biofilm itself is microscopic.

30 *Correct answer A*: It is the toxins produced by the anaerobic bacteria that attack the alveolar bone and cause gradual tooth mobility, rather than the microorganisms themselves. All three of the other options are true statements.

Scientific Principles in the Management of Oral Health Diseases and Dental Procedures

Understand the Methods for the Prevention and Management of Oral Diseases

Questions

1 Which one of the following disease processes presents as a slow-growing abnormal sac of fluid within the body tissues?
   A Benign tumour
   B Cyst
   C Infection
   D Ulcer

2 There are three main areas of caries prevention available to the patient and the dental team. Which one of the following areas is not relevant to caries prevention?
   A Control the build-up of plaque
   B Control the host response
   C Increase tooth resistance to acid attack
   D Modify the diet

3 Which one of the following toothpaste ingredients has the most effect on suppressing the formation of plaque?
   A Biological enzymes
   B Sodium fluoride
   C Sodium saccharin
   D Triclosan

Questions and Answers for Diploma in Dental Nursing, Level 3, First Edition. Carole Hollins.
© 2016 John Wiley & Sons, Ltd. Published 2016 by John Wiley & Sons, Ltd.

4 Patients should be taught good oral hygiene techniques by members of the dental team. Which one of the following actions should patients not be instructed to carry out while receiving toothbrushing instructions?

A Brush for at least 2 min

B Brush twice daily

C Rinse out after brushing

D Use fluoridated toothpaste

5 The enamel surface of a tooth can be destroyed by factors other than dental caries. Which one of the following terms is used to describe buccal enamel loss due to mechanical trauma from toothbrushing?

A Abfraction

B Abrasion

C Attrition

D Erosion

6 Which one of the following areas in the oral cavity is least effectively cleaned by manual toothbrushing?

A Gingival crevice

B Interdental area

C Lingual tooth surface

D Occlusal fissure

7 Which one of the following disease processes presents as a localised swelling, often with pus present?

A Cyst

B Infection

C Malignant tumour

D Ulcer

8 Mouthwashes contain a variety of ingredients depending on the reason for the particular use of each one. Which one of the following ingredients is added specifically to aid healing by the elimination of anaerobic bacteria?

A Chlorhexidine

B Hydrogen peroxide

C Sodium fluoride

D Triclosan

9 Which one of the following statements about fluoride is false?

A Fluorapatite crystals make enamel more resistant to acid attack

B Fluoridation of water is an example of topical fluoride application

C Fluoride replaces hydroxyapatite crystals in the enamel

D Fluoride slows down the feeding rate of oral bacteria

10 Which one of the following periodontal conditions may be caused by bacterial infection with *Treponema vincenti*?

   A Acute herpetic gingivitis
   B Acute lateral periodontal abscess
   C Acute necrotising ulcerative gingivitis
   D Subacute pericoronitis

11 Which one of the following oral hygiene products is the least effective in removing plaque from between tooth contact points?

   A Floss
   B Interdental brush
   C Tape
   D Woodstick

12 Which one of the following disease processes presents as an overgrowth of tissue cells that invade their surroundings and often destroy those surrounding tissues?

   A Cyst
   B Infection
   C Tumour
   D Ulcer

13 Detergent foods are those recommended to be eaten after a meal to remove loose food debris and reduce the risk of caries, when conventional oral hygiene methods are unable to be carried out. Which one of the following is a detergent food in this context?

   A Carrot
   B Cracker
   C Grapes
   D Yoghurt

14 Which one of the following options is an example of a systemic fluoride application?

   A Fluoride drops
   B Fluoride mouthwash
   C Fluoride toothpaste
   D Fluoride varnish

15 One method of determining the effect of varying social factors on oral health in a population is to measure the DMF levels of that population. Which of the following is the correct meaning of DMF?

   A Decayed, missing and filled
   B Decayed, missing and fluoridated
   C Diseased, missing and filled
   D Diseased, missing and fluoridated

16 Which one of the following options listed is the main aim of good communication between the dental team and the patient, in relation to their oral health?
   A To determine their frequency of brushing
   B To determine their level of motivation
   C To discover the oral health products they use
   D To make friends with the patient

17 Which one of the following risk factors for general poor health is also associated with enamel erosion of the teeth?
   A Alcoholism
   B Bulimia
   C Obesity
   D Smoking

18 Which one of the following toothpaste ingredients has the most effect on increasing the teeth's resistance to caries?
   A Biological enzymes
   B Sodium fluoride
   C Sodium saccharin
   D Triclosan

19 Many sugars added to carbohydrate foods cause dental caries. Which one of the following sugars is not associated with dental caries?
   A Dextrose
   B Glucose
   C Lactose
   D Sucrose

20 There are many contributory factors associated with the worsening of a periodontal condition that is already present in a patient. Which one of the following statements is true with regard to potential contributory factors?
   A Hormonal imbalance during puberty has no effect on periodontal health
   B Medication prescribed for epilepsy causes gingival hyperplasia
   C Nicotine products in cigarettes cause gingival bleeding
   D Use of non-fluoride toothpastes is associated with periodontal disease

21 The enamel may be lost from a tooth due to factors other than dental caries. Which one of the following describes enamel loss due to the action of dietary acids?
   A Abfraction
   B Abrasion
   C Attrition
   D Erosion

22 Which one of the following disease processes presents as a break in the protective layer of a soft tissue, leaving a raw and often painful lesion that may bleed?

A Benign tumour

B Cyst

C Infection

D Ulcer

23 Which one of the following is an example of a systemic fluoride oral health product?

A Fluoride gel

B Fluoride mouthwash

C Fluoride tablet

D Fluoride toothpaste

24 Which one of the following toothpaste ingredients has the most effect on removing some surface stains from the teeth?

A Biological enzymes

B Sodium fluoride

C Sodium saccharin

D Triclosan

25 An oral health assessment is carried out when a patient attends the dental workplace. Which one of the following options states information that is required by the dental team to be able to determine the likely success of any oral health promotion efforts?

A Employment details

B Known risk factors

C Preferred recall interval

D Previous dental provider

26 Which one of the following is the ideal concentration of fluoride that is artificially added to water supplies as a public health measure, in parts per million (ppm)?

A 0.1 ppm

B 1 ppm

C 10 ppm

D 100 ppm

27 There are three main areas of control and prevention of periodontal disease available to the patient and the dental team. Which one of the following areas is not relevant to the control and prevention of periodontal disease?

A Control the build-up of plaque

B Control the host response

C Modify the contributory factors

D Modify the diet

28 Which one of the following actions describes the best method of reinforcing the oral health advice given to a patient at the end of an appointment, so that they remember the details?

A Ask the receptionist to reiterate it

B Give it in writing

C Repeat it before they leave

D Repeat it at the next appointment

29 Known risk factors relating to poor oral health are often found to relate to poor general health too. Which one of the following general health conditions is not necessarily associated with poor oral health?

A Bulimia

B Diabetes

C Hypertension

D Smoking-related respiratory disease

30 Good communication skills are important in encouraging patients to help to manage their own oral health. Which one of the following indicates a dismissive attitude towards the patient when carried out during an oral health discussion?

A Butting in verbally

B Folding the arms

C Sitting down

D Turning away

31 Various prescribed medicines have side effects that may affect the oral health of the patient. Which one of the following types of medicine is known to reduce salivary flow in patients, so that they develop a dry mouth?

A Analgesics

B Anti-epileptics

C Diuretics

D Immunosuppressants

32 Dietary analysis often reveals that patients consume food and drinks containing hidden sugars. Which one of the following statements about hidden sugars is false?

A Added by manufacturer during processing

B Have an effect on caries rate

C Added to make foods taste sweet

D Often found in low-fat products

Answers

1 *Correct answer B*: Dental examples include the dentigerous cyst, which grows around the crown of an unerupted tooth, especially molars. A benign tumour is a harmless overgrowth of tissue, an infection occurs as a localised swelling with pus present, and an ulcer occurs as a break in the protective tissue layer (skin or mucous membrane) that leaves a raw and often painful lesion.

2 *Correct answer B*: The response of the tooth to attack by caries cannot be altered or controlled – a cavity will form. Plaque build-up can be controlled by good oral hygiene efforts, tooth resistance can be increased with the use of fluoride products, and the diet can be modified to reduce the amount and frequency of consumption of cariogenic foods and drinks.

3 *Correct answer D*: This is the active ingredient in toothpastes aimed specifically at fighting 'gum disease' rather than caries, by suppressing the formation of plaque in the mouth. Biological enzymes are included to assist in stain removal in various 'whitening' products, sodium fluoride is the standard ingredient of most toothpastes that is added to increase the tooth's resistance to acid attack, and sodium saccharin is added to give a pleasant taste to the product.

4 *Correct answer C*: Rinsing out after toothbrushing will immediately remove the fluoridated toothpaste from the mouth – this should be left to bathe the teeth and allow maximum absorption of the fluoride content into the teeth as a topical fluoride product. All three of the other options are correct.

5 *Correct answer B*: A horizontal groove is gradually worn into the buccal and labial surfaces of the teeth by the sawing action of the toothbrush during brushing by a heavy-handed patient. The class V appearance of the non-carious cavity that is created can be responsible for severe sensitivity in the teeth affected.

6 *Correct answer B*: The toothbrush bristles are too large to enter and clean the contact point area of the teeth effectively, unless the patient has natural or extraction gaps between their teeth. All three of the other areas can be adequately cleaned using a manual toothbrush.

7 *Correct answer B*: This is a classic appearance of an infection. A cyst presents as an abnormal, fluid-filled sac; an ulcer presents as a shallow breach in the skin or mucous membrane with a raw, painful base; and a malignant tumour can appear in any guise. An abnormal tissue appearance that fails to heal and resolve after normal efforts to treat the presenting lesion should determine the need for further investigation.

8 *Correct answer B*: Hydrogen peroxide products fizz and effervesce when swilled around the mouth, creating lots of oxygen bubbles that help to kill anaerobic bacteria (those that thrive in low-oxygen levels). These types of bacteria are found in wounds and in diseased periodontal tissues, and the mouthwash is particularly useful to aid healing after surgery, trauma and acute infections of deeper tissues and to help resolve painful lesions such as aphthous ulcers.

9 *Correct answer B*: Water fluoridation is an example of systemic fluoride, where the fluoridated product is taken internally rather than applied externally to the teeth, as would a topical fluoride product. All three of the other options are true.

10 *Correct answer C*: Acute necrotising ulcerative gingivitis, also used to be known as Vincent's gingivitis, is an acute periodontal infection involving the named spirochaete, which is often seen in teenagers and young adults with poor oral hygiene, especially in those who also smoke.

11 *Correct answer D*: Woodsticks cannot be angled or wrapped around the tooth to provide good tooth contact as the other products can, and generally, they just push solid food debris from between the teeth without having any tooth cleaning effect.

12 *Correct answer C*: Of the options listed, only a tumour involves the overgrowth of tissue cells. Benign tumours tend to push other tissues apart, but the sinister nature of a malignant tumour is in part due to its habit of invading and destroying surrounding tissues, making the damage it causes very difficult (or impossible) to treat in some cases.

13 *Correct answer A*: The crunchy nature of the carrot will dislodge food debris, and the vegetable contains no non-milk extrinsic sugar. Grapes are too soft to have the same effect, and crackers and yoghurt may both contain hidden sugars, as well as being too soft to dislodge food debris.

14 *Correct answer A:* A systemic fluoride is one that is ingested to allow its internal incorporation into the tooth structure, whereas topical fluorides are those applied externally to the outer surface of the tooth. Only fluoride drops are taken internally; all three of the other options are examples of topical fluorides.

15 *Correct answer A*: The DMF is a score of the numbers of teeth of a patient that show signs of carious attack, removal by extraction or dental intervention to treat previous caries – the higher the scores, the poorer the oral health of the individual.

16 *Correct answer B*: The level of motivation that a patient has with regard to their oral health and maintaining or improving it will determine the level of advice, support and treatment that the patient receives from the dental team. This cannot be realised without having a good rapport and good communication with the patient. Some patients are not interested in their oral health and do not wish to be constantly advised on how to improve it (that is their right), and they are likely to become irritated at being bombarded with oral health information at each attendance. On the other hand, some patients are keen to be advised and supported by the dental team but will only feel comfortable about asking for help if the team are friendly and approachable and have good communication skills. All of the other three options will be realised once oral health advice is being discussed.

17 *Correct answer B*: Sufferers of this emotional disorder induce self-vomiting in an effort to control or reduce their weight, and the recurrent acidic vomit causes characteristic enamel erosion of their teeth. All three of the other options are not specifically associated with acid erosion of the teeth. Alcoholism and smoking are associated with an increased instance of oral cancer, and obesity may be linked with a high rate of caries due to the types of foods and drinks that are consumed.

18 *Correct answer B*: Sodium fluoride is added to the vast majority of oral health products to provide topical fluoride to the teeth on each use. The fluoride becomes incorporated into the crystalline hydroxyapatite structure of the enamel, making it stronger and more able to resist demineralisation by dietary acids.

19 *Correct answer C*: This is a naturally occurring sugar found in milk that produces so little organic acid that it is considered harmless to teeth – it is a milk extrinsic sugar. All three of the other options are cariogenic. Dextrose and sucrose are refined, non-milk extrinsic sugars, and glucose can occur naturally but may also be refined and will act as a non-milk extrinsic sugar.

20 *Correct answer B*: The drug phenytoin (Epanutin) has the side effect of causing gingival hyperplasia so that affected patients appear with generalised false pockets. Hormonal imbalance during puberty is linked with poor periodontal health, specifically acute necrotising ulcerative gingivitis. Nicotine products actually reduce gingival bleeding, making periodontal problems more difficult to diagnose. Fluoride has no effect on the prevalence of periodontal disease.

21 *Correct answer D*: Enamel loss due to dietary acids occurs in a typical pattern, affecting the labial surfaces of the upper anterior teeth and the occlusal surfaces of the posterior teeth. It is called erosion and may result in severe tooth sensitivity as the enamel is lost and the underlying dentine becomes exposed.

22 *Correct answer D*: This is the typical appearance of an ulcer, although those associated with sinister lesions such as squamous cell carcinoma tend to be painless and do not resolve when obvious causes have been removed.

23 *Correct answer C*: Systemic fluorides are those that are ingested in some form, such as a fluoride tablet. Topical fluorides are applied to the external surface of the teeth and are not ingested. All three of the other options are examples of topical fluorides.

24 *Correct answer A*: Biological enzymes have replaced abrasive products in toothpastes and are added to remove surface staining from the teeth. This reveals the actual colour of the teeth, although the majority of the products are sold as 'whitening' agents. Triclosan is added to suppress the production of plaque in the mouth and therefore reduce the amount of tartar that builds up.

25 *Correct answer B*: Risk factors associated with caries incidence and periodontal disease prevalence need to be identified before relevant oral health promotion and instruction can be given. Patients with diets high in cariogenic foods and acid drinks need to be identified before relevant diet and oral health product information can be given. Similarly, smokers, diabetics and other 'at-risk' patients of periodontal disease need to be identified before relevant oral hygiene instruction and lifestyle information can be given. Some information will be provided during the completion of medical history questionnaires; other points may need to be specifically discussed.

26 *Correct answer B*: This is the ideal concentration of systemic fluoride to be incorporated into water supplies that contain no fluoride to give the maximum caries prevention without causing enamel fluorosis. Lower concentrations will be ineffective at reducing caries incidence, while higher levels are likely to cause enamel fluorosis – an unsightly mottling of the tooth enamel due to high fluoride intake.

27 *Correct answer D*: A patient's diet has no influence on their periodontal disease experience, but is hugely significant to their caries experience.

28 *Correct answer B*: Written information can be taken away by the patient and read at a later date without that information having to be remembered. All three of the other options require the patient to remember verbal information that they have been told by the dental team. This is likely to be forgotten not long after the patient leaves the premises and will therefore have little impact on their oral health routine.

29 *Correct answer C*: Hypertension (high blood pressure) is not directly associated with poor oral health; the disease has no oral manifestations that will aid diagnosis, nor does the condition affect the oral tissues detrimentally. Bulimic patients will have signs of acid erosion on their teeth, diabetics will exhibit poor wound healing and an exacerbation of any periodontal disease they have, and smokers will tend to have stained teeth, exacerbated periodontal disease and possibly various oral soft tissue lesions that may be premalignant or malignant.

30 *Correct answer D*: This is a classic act of using body language to dismiss someone, indicating a lack of interest by the listener in the patient. Butting in while the patient is talking is rude and overbearing, but is not dismissive as it happens during the discussion. Folded arms indicate defensiveness – as though the listener has something to hide – while sitting down during a discussion indicates an interest in what the patient is saying and a willingness to take part in the discussion.

31 *Correct answer C*: Diuretics (often referred to as 'water tablets') are given to patients with heart disease to reduce the excess fluid load on their heart, so that it is not under strain while pumping the blood around the body. The excess fluid is urinated out by the patient, but the drug has a water-reducing effect on all other relevant tissues, including the salivary glands. The patients therefore often complain of a dry mouth. All three of the other options have no effect on the salivary glands.

32 *Correct answer C*: Although some foods may taste sweet due to their hidden sugar content, it is added to other foods merely to assist in the manufacturing process, with no effect on taste. Tomato soup and ketchup, for example, both contain hidden sugars, but neither product could be described as anything other than savoury.

OUTCOME 3

Know How to Manage and Handle Materials and Instruments during Dental Procedures

Questions

1 The dentist may use various items during the preparation of a cavity to receive an amalgam restoration. Which one of the following options is used to provide the best tactile sensation during cavity preparation?

A Air turbine with diamond bur
B Double-ended amalgam plugger
C Double-ended excavator
D Slow-speed handpiece with stainless steel bur

2 Which one of the following moisture control techniques is the most successful at preventing tooth contamination during endodontic treatment?

A Cotton wool rolls
B High-speed suction
C Low-speed suction
D Rubber dam

3 The vast majority of dental procedures are carried out under local anaesthetic so that the patient feels no pain. Which one of the following constituents of a local anaesthetic cartridge is present to maintain a neutral pH of 7, so that the solution does not irritate the soft tissues?

A Anaesthetic
B Buffer
C Preservative
D Vasoconstrictor

Questions and Answers for Diploma in Dental Nursing, Level 3, First Edition. Carole Hollins.
© 2016 John Wiley & Sons, Ltd. Published 2016 by John Wiley & Sons, Ltd.

4 Which one of the following hand instruments is most likely to be used to place and contour composite filling material into an anterior tooth cavity?

A Amalgam plugger

B Ball-ended burnisher

C Excavator

D Flat plastic

5 Which one of the following restorative materials is not suitable for use as a temporary filling in a deciduous tooth?

A Calcium hydroxide

B Glass ionomer

C Zinc phosphate

D Zinc polycarboxylate

6 Which one of the following is the correct classification of a mesio-palatal cavity in the upper right lateral incisor?

A Class I

B Class II

C Class III

D Class IV

7 What is the purpose of using local anaesthetic equipment capable of aspiration when administering anaesthetic to a patient?

A Allows a painless technique

B Allows a rapid technique

C Avoids injection into a blood vessel

D Avoids injection into the nerve trunk

8 Which one of the following options describes the most likely use of a spoon excavator during dental procedures?

A Remove loose crowns

B Remove softened dentine

C Remove unsupported enamel

D Retract soft tissues

9 Which one of the following instruments is specifically used to remove calculus from the interproximal areas of teeth?

A Jacquette scaler

B Push scaler

C Sickle scaler

D Ultrasonic scaler

10 Which one of the following options is not a typical use of a mouth mirror during dental procedures?

   A Aid vision

   B Detect overhangs

   C Reflect light

   D Retract tissues

11 Which one of the following options is the description of a class V cavity in a tooth?

   A Involves a single surface in a pit or fissure

   B Involves the cervical margin of a tooth

   C Involves the mesial surface of an incisor

   D Involves two surfaces of a posterior tooth

12 Which one of the following items is correctly used to extirpate the pulp contents during endodontic treatment?

   A Barbed broach

   B Finger spreader

   C Gates Glidden drill

   D Hand file

13 Which one of the following options is the correct category of waste disposal for a used local anaesthetic cartridge?

   A Infectious hazardous waste – sharps

   B Infectious hazardous waste – soft

   C Non-hazardous waste

   D Non-infectious hazardous waste – chemical

14 Dental burs are used for a variety of reasons during dental procedures. Which one of the following bur shapes is most likely to be used during an inlay preparation to ensure no undercuts are produced?

   A Flat fissure

   B Pear

   C Round

   D Tapered fissure

15 Which one of the following hand instruments is usually used to adapt a filling material to the cavity margins to avoid leakage under the set restoration?

   A Amalgam plugger

   B Burnisher

   C Flat plastic

   D Spoon excavator

16 Which one of the following rubber dam kit items is used to hold the dam sheet in place around a tooth during dental procedures?

A Clamp

B Forceps

C Frame

D Punch

17 Zinc oxide and eugenol cement has many uses in dentistry. Which one of the following situations is one where this material would not be used?

A Impression paste

B Lining under composite

C Periodontal dressing

D Root filling paste

18 Many partial dentures are designed with metal clasps to aid their retention. Which one of the following methods provides the natural retention of an upper full denture?

A Adhesive paste

B Muscle contractions

C Suction pads

D Surface tension

19 A spillage of mercury has occurred that requires the use of the mercury spillage kit. Which one of the following options is the first action to be taken when dealing with the spillage?

A Apply personal protective equipment

B Apply the paste to the spillage

C Mix the mercury-absorbent paste

D Vacuum the area

20 The vast majority of dental procedures are carried out under local anaesthetic so that the patient feels no pain. Which one of the following constituents of a local anaesthetic cartridge is present to allow a reasonable shelf life and period of use?

A Anaesthetic

B Buffer

C Preservative

D Vasoconstrictor

21 Various matrix systems are available for use during tooth restoration to ensure that filling materials remain in the cavity during setting. Which one of the following types of matrix system is most likely to be used when placing a composite filling in a class III cavity?

A Cervical foil

B Plastic

    C Siqveland

    D Tofflemire

22 During which procedure might a Willis bite gauge be required?

    A Bite recording of full dentures

    B Implant assessment

    C Occlusal recording of four-unit bridge

    D Orthodontic overbite measurement

23 Which one of the following metals makes up the largest proportion of alloy powder in the restorative material amalgam?

    A Copper

    B Silver

    C Tin

    D Zinc

24 Which type of local anaesthetic administration technique involves depositing the anaesthetic solution beneath the mucous membrane and over the alveolar bone to anaesthetise the local nerve endings?

    A Infiltration

    B Intra-ligamentary

    C Intra-osseous

    D Nerve block

25 Before taking an impression of a crown preparation, the margins of the tooth must be made clearly visible. Which one of the following items is used to achieve this?

    A Crown form

    B Matrix band

    C Retraction cord

    D Wooden wedge

26 Which one of the following materials is acidic and may cause pulpal irritation in deep cavities?

    A Calcium hydroxide paste

    B Glass ionomer cement

    C Zinc phosphate cement

    D Zinc polycarboxylate cement

27 Which one of the following options is the description of a class III cavity in a tooth?

    A Involves a single surface in a pit or fissure

    B Involves the cervical margin of a tooth

    C Involves the mesial surface of an incisor

    D Involves two surfaces of a posterior tooth

28 When is it unlikely that a pair of Adams pliers will be required at an orthodontic appointment?

   A Adjusting a functional appliance
   B Debonding a fixed appliance
   C Fitting a removable appliance
   D Tightening a removable retainer

29 Which one of the following temporary filling materials is most adhesive to the dentine surface of the cavity?

   A Gutta-percha as greenstick
   B Zinc oxide and eugenol cement
   C Zinc phosphate cement
   D Zinc polycarboxylate cement

30 When a fixed prosthesis is to be constructed, the technician is provided with an impression of the dental arch containing the prepared tooth. Which one of the following materials will not be used for this impression?

   A Addition silicone
   B Alginate
   C Polyether
   D Polyvinyl siloxane

31 Which one of the following options is not a usual route of entry into the body by mercury when mercury poisoning has occurred?

   A Absorption
   B Ingestion
   C Inhalation
   D Inoculation

32 Which one of the following medical conditions is likely to dictate the use of a local anaesthetic without adrenaline present as a vasoconstrictor?

   A Hypertension
   B Hypoglycaemia
   C Hypothyroidism
   D Pregnancy

33 Which one of the following is the correct constitution of acid etchant that is used during a restorative procedure using composite material?

   A 10% hydrochloric acid
   B 25% polyacrylic acid
   C 33% phosphoric acid
   D 46% hydrogen peroxide

34 Which one of the following properties is an additional advantage that calcium hydroxide has over other lining materials?

A Chemically calms the pulp

B Promotes the formation of secondary dentine

C Protects the pulp from chemical irritation

D Seals the pulp from residual bacteria

35 Which type of local anaesthetic administration technique involves depositing the anaesthetic solution directly into the cancellous layer of the alveolar bone to anaesthetise the tooth roots?

A Infiltration

B Intra-ligamentary

C Intra-osseous

D Nerve block

36 What is the correct category of waste disposal for an extracted tooth containing an amalgam filling?

A Infectious (clinical) sharps

B Non-hazardous waste

C Non-infectious (chemical)

D Offensive waste

37 A curing light is often used to set modern composite filling materials. Which one of the following indicates the accepted depth to which these lights can penetrate the restoration?

A 1.0 mm

B 1.5 mm

C 2.0 mm

D 2.5 mm

38 Which one of the following is the first action that must be carried out to an alginate impression that has just been removed from the patient's mouth in an effort to render it safe to be handled by the laboratory staff?

A Cover with damp gauze to prevent it drying out

B Immerse in a chemical bath to disinfect it

C Rinse under running water to remove gross debris

D Spray with a disinfectant to decontaminate it

39 Which one of the following devices allows aspirated waste amalgam residue to be collected and safely disposed of by the dental team before it is able to enter the drains?

A Amalgam separator

B Amalgam trap

C Mercury spillage kit

D Reverse osmosis machine

40 The vast majority of dental procedures are carried out under local anaesthetic so that the patient feels no pain. Which one of the following constituents of a local anaesthetic cartridge is present to prolong the action of the anaesthetic?

   A Anaesthetic

   B Buffer

   C Preservative

   D Vasoconstrictor

41 Glass ionomer cements are a widely used dental material. Which one of the following options states the main advantage of this material over composites?

   A Adhesive to enamel

   B Easily polished

   C Releases fluoride

   D Superior strength

42 Which one of the following options is the description of a class II cavity in a tooth?

   A Involves a single surface in a pit or fissure

   B Involves the cervical margin of a tooth

   C Involves the mesial surface of an incisor

   D Involves two surfaces of a posterior tooth

43 Which one of the following is the correct action to take following a small spillage of mercury in the dental workplace?

   A Collect globules into the waste pot

   B Cover the spillage with sodium hypochlorite

   C Report to the Health and Safety Executive

   D Vacuum the area thoroughly

44 Which one of the following terms is used to describe an endodontic technique of removing contaminated pulp tissue from the pulp chamber only, leaving that in the root canal intact?

   A Apicoectomy

   B Pulp capping

   C Pulpectomy

   D Pulpotomy

45 Which one of the following impression materials must be stored in a damp state once it has been used to take an impression to prevent distortion?

   A Addition silicone

   B Alginate

   C Polyether

   D Polyvinyl siloxane

46 Which of the following examples of a fixed prosthodontic device is the term used to describe one used to restore a cavity in a tooth?

A Bridge

B Crown

C Inlay

D Veneer

47 Mercury poisoning may occur after exposure to small amounts of the chemical over long periods of time. Which one of the following body organs can be irreparably damaged by mercury?

A Brain

B Kidney

C Lung

D Stomach

48 Which one of the following components of a fixed orthodontic appliance may be used to hold the archwire in place on molar teeth during treatment?

A Alastik (module)

B Bracket

C Elastic

D Tube

49 During an extraction procedure, it may be necessary to remove sharp spicules of the bone from the dental ridge to allow full healing to occur. Which one of the following instruments may be used to carry out this task?

A Dissecting forceps

B Mosquito forceps

C Osteotrimmer

D Rongeurs

50 Missing teeth may be replaced in several ways. Which one of the following devices is not a recognised method of replacing missing teeth?

A Bridge

B Denture

C Functional appliance

D Implant

51 Which one of the following luting cements acts by being mechanically adhesive to the rough inner surface of a crown or bridge and the tooth?

A Glass ionomer cement

B Self-cure resin

C Zinc phosphate cement

D Zinc polycarboxylate cement

52 Which one of the following chemical compounds from the mercury spillage kit is mixed with flowers of sulphur and water to make the paste used to contain a mercury spillage?

A Calcium hydroxide

B Calcium sulphate

C Phosphoric acid

D Sodium hypochlorite

53 Which type of local anaesthetic administration technique will usually require the use of an aspirating syringe and appropriate cartridge, with a long 27 gauge needle?

A Infiltration of upper molars

B Intra-ligamentary of lower molars

C Intra-osseous of upper molars

D Nerve block of lower molars

54 During a root filling procedure, the root canal is widened in its natural shape by the use of instruments to clean and debride its walls. Which one of the following instruments is used to carry out this stage of treatment?

A File

B Finger plugger

C Plain broach

D Reamer

55 Which of the following statements about immediate replacement dentures is false?

A Can replace more than one tooth

B May require replacement within 6 months

C Require impression to be constructed

D Require try-in stage

Answers

1 *Correct answer C*: All hand instruments will give better tactile sensation (touch) than either of the handpieces, as these are power operated and run with a vibratory action. The excavator is used specifically to scrape the cavity base and walls and spoon out any remaining softened dentine after the majority of the cavity has been prepared using the air turbine and then the slow-speed handpiece. The amalgam plugger is used to firmly press the amalgam into the cavity during filling.

2 *Correct answer D*: Rubber dam physically isolates the tooth under treatment from the rest of the mouth, so it does not become contaminated by saliva or any bacteria in the mouth while the procedure is undertaken. With endodontic treatment, this is particularly important, as the pulp chamber of the tooth is open and any bacterial contamination can enter here and potentially pass through the tooth apex into the deeper tissues. Unless the contamination is removed, the treatment may fail.

3 *Correct answer B*: If the cartridge contents are acidic (pH below 7), then the buffer constituent is added by the manufacturers to ensure that it is neutralised and the pH is raised to 7. If the cartridge contents are alkaline (pH above 7), then the buffer constituent is added to neutralise the solution so that the pH is lowered to 7. The anaesthetic constituent acts on the nerves to produce numbness, the preservative prevents the solution from deteriorating and 'going off', and the vasoconstrictor prolongs the working time of the anaesthetic by closing down the local blood vessels.

4 *Correct answer D*: This is the main use of the flat plastic instrument. Their ends can also be gently curved to provide even better contouring of the composite material, which is especially useful when the rounded shape of the tooth is being imitated. Burnishers are used to smooth the filling surface (especially amalgam) and adapt it to the cavity margins.

5 *Correct answer A*: Calcium hydroxide is used in a paste consistency to line cavities. It is not thick and bulky enough to be built up into a temporary filling in any tooth. All three of the other options are suitable materials to be used as temporary fillings.

6 *Correct answer C*: A class III cavity is defined as one that affects two or more surfaces of an anterior tooth. If the same cavity included the incisal edge of the tooth as well, it would be a class IV cavity.

7 *Correct answer C*: Many anaesthetics contain the vasoconstrictor adrenaline to prolong the working time of the solution. If adrenaline is accidentally injected into a blood vessel during anaesthesia, it will act as a strong heart stimulant and cause palpitations. In patients with heart disease, this may be dangerous to them. During the aspirating technique, the needle is positioned and then the plunger is pulled back before injection. If the needle tip is in a blood vessel, blood will visibly pool into the cartridge – the needle tip can then be safely repositioned before the injection is given.

8 *Correct answer B*: Once a cavity has been accessed and the majority of the caries has been removed using handpieces and burs, the operator resorts to the use of hand instruments to complete caries removal while avoiding breaching the pulp chamber. The spoon excavator is the usual instrument to carry out this process – its sharp edges are able to scrape over and scoop out any softened dentine in a controlled manner, and the change to hard dentine once caries removal is complete can be felt while using the instrument.

9 *Correct answer B*: The flat blade design of this scaler is pushed between the teeth to dislodge supragingival calculus present in the interproximal areas, usually of the lower anterior teeth. The Jaquette and sickle scalers do not have flat blades to be used in this way. Ultrasonic scalers have various tip shapes available, but not specifically for use in the interproximal areas.

10 *Correct answer B*: Overhangs on fillings tend to occur interproximally, where vision is limited during the restorative procedure. They are more easily detected using a probe to catch on the edge of the overhanging filling or are clearly seen on radiographs, especially bitewings. All three of the other options are typical uses of the mouth mirror.

11 *Correct answer B*: Class V cavities may occur on any tooth, but they always involve the cervical margin (the neck) of the tooth. A typical abrasion cavity that has been caused by vigorous sawing actions during toothbrushing will appear as a class V cavity, or they occur by poor toothbrushing of the gingival margins so that a carious cavity forms.

12 *Correct answer A*: The barbs along the end section of the broach engage the soft tissue of the pulp as the instrument is twisted in the root canal, pulling the pulp out as the instrument is removed. A Gates Glidden drill is used by some dentists to access the pulp chamber and drill out its contents in one action, but this is not the designated use of these drills.

13 *Correct answer A*: The local anaesthetic cartridges are made of glass or plastic, both of which may cause a sharps injury to someone if they shatter or break. Therefore, they must be safely disposed of in the rigid sharps container, along with needles, hand files, matrix bands and any other sharp items.

14 *Correct answer D*: The bur is tapered from its base (the end that engages the handpiece) towards its tip so that a very slight deviation from parallel is produced when a tooth is prepared using the bur. This prevents undercuts being introduced into the preparation but gives the most retentive shape to the inlay cavity. Pear and round burs will both produce undercuts as will a flat fissure bur if it is not held exactly parallel to the tooth during use.

15 *Correct answer B*: Although originally intended to burnish thin edges of gold to the tooth surface, burnishers are useful instruments to adapt amalgam and other plastic materials to the cavity margins before setting. Flat plastic instruments are more useful for contouring materials.

16 *Correct answer A*: The rubber dam clamps are provided in a range of sizes and shapes to fit around individual teeth – small and large molars, premolars and anterior tooth clamps (also called butterfly clamps). They are placed using the clamp forceps once the dam is in place over the tooth, and when released from the forceps, they grip tightly around the neck of the tooth so that the dam sheet is held firmly in place.

17 *Correct answer B*: The oily eugenol liquid reacts adversely with composite materials and prevents them from fully setting, making zinc oxide and eugenol cement unsuitable as a lining beneath these restorations. All three of the other options are uses of proprietary brands of the cement.

18 *Correct answer D*: The layer of saliva that lies trapped beneath the palate of the upper full denture allows the surface tension of the fluid to act in a retentive manner, holding the denture up. Although some patients use adhesive pastes to improve the retention of their denture, a well-fitting one should not require their regular use. Muscle contractions help to retain a denture by holding the flanges in the sulci, but suction pads are not used for denture retention.

19 *Correct answer A*: Mercury is poisonous and can gain entry to the body by ingestion, inhalation of the vapours or absorption through the skin and mucous membranes. The application of full PPE before dealing with a spillage will protect the staff member from mercury poisoning. A spillage should never be vacuumed as this increases the level of mercury vapour in the air and makes poisoning by inhalation more likely.

20 *Correct answer C*: As with all other drugs and materials, the constituents within a local anaesthetic cartridge will deteriorate with time so that they become ineffective or even dangerous to use, if they break down with age into other chemicals. A preservative is added to slow down this deterioration and allow a reasonable period of use before the cartridge has to be discarded – this is called its 'shelf life', and the point at which it should no longer be used is called its expiry date.

21 *Correct answer B*: The vast majority of composite materials available today are those that set by light cure. The blue light must be able to penetrate the material to cause it to set, so only a plastic matrix can be used as the light can pass through this. A cervical foil matrix is used for glass ionomer restorations in class V cavities, and both Siqveland and Tofflemire are metal matrix systems for use on posterior teeth with amalgam restorations.

22 *Correct answer A*: The gauge is used to measure the occlusal face height of the patient, so that the dentures constructed will allow sufficient mouth opening. The top is positioned under the patient's nose and the moveable bottom section is slid up or down the gauge until it rests beneath their chin. The patient is then guided to open or close their mouth by the dentist until a suitable position is found where the patient is comfortable and the mouth position is not straining their muscles. The slider is then locked in at this point, and the position is measured on the gauge as a length in mm. With this known measurement, the technician will then construct the try-ins of the dentures so that the patient has a comfortable and functional face height.

23 *Correct answer B*: Silver is present in alloy powder in quantities of between 70 and 75% of the total alloy powder. Copper quantities are much less and are varied to provide a range of amalgam products that are described as regular or high-copper alloys, while tin and zinc are present in very small amounts.

24 *Correct answer A*: Infiltration can be used to anaesthetise any tooth or soft tissue where their nerve supply lies outside the alveolar bone of the jaws or outside the palatal bones in the roof of the mouth. Therefore, the lower molar, premolar and canine teeth are the only ones that cannot be anaesthetised by infiltration. The molars require an inferior dental nerve block technique, while the premolars and canine require a mental nerve block (although the inferior dental nerve block will anaesthetise all the lower teeth). In the upper jaw, a posterior superior dental nerve block can be used for the second and third molars if necessary, but they can also be anaesthetised by buccal infiltration.

25 *Correct answer C*: The cord is soaked in a haemostat such as adrenaline and then pushed into the gingival crevice to cause tissue shrinkage immediately around the prepared tooth. It is removed from the crevice just before the impression is taken, so that the gingival tissues are clear of the preparation margins and the technician is able to construct a well-fitting crown.

26 *Correct answer C*: The liquid component of zinc phosphate cement is phosphoric acid with a pH of 2. When initially mixed and placed, the unset cement will therefore be very acidic, and it should be used as a temporary filling or a base with great care in deep cavities and in deciduous teeth, where the pulp tissues lie close to the cavity surface. Calcium hydroxide is a suitable liner to be placed beneath the base to protect the pulp, or either of the other two options can be used as an alternative material.

27 *Correct answer C*: A class III cavity always involves anterior teeth rather than posterior teeth, and it may be a mesial or distal surface that is involved. The cavity may also extend to include the labial, lingual or palatal surface of the tooth and still be classified as a class III cavity, but once the incisal edge becomes involved, the cavity is described as class IV.

28 *Correct answer B*: Bracket and band removers will be required for this procedure. Adams pliers are used to adjust the stainless steel components of removable and functional appliances, as well as those used to retain removable retainers.

29 *Correct answer D*: Superior adhesion to dentine makes zinc polycarboxylate the best material to be used as a luting cement of the older types of materials available. Modern dual-cure materials are better still as they tend not to dissolve in saliva over time like the older materials, resulting in the eventual loss of the fixed prosthesis from the tooth.

30 *Correct answer B*: Alginate is not sufficiently accurate to be used for fixed prosthetic impressions, and it also tears easily compared to the elastomer materials. All three of the other options are elastomer materials that are used for fixed prosthetic impressions.

31 *Correct answer D*: Entry by inoculation would require the mercury to be injected into the person. All three of the other options are known methods of entry for mercury and its vapours.

32 *Correct answer A*: Adrenaline is a cardiac stimulant that acts to increase the rate and depth of the heartbeat. Patients with hypertension (high blood pressure) have some level of cardiovascular disease that is causing the heart to overwork, resulting in a raised blood pressure. Adrenaline in local anaesthetic would cause a higher pressure still, with possibly serious medical consequences.

33 *Correct answer C*: Phosphoric acid is supplied in both gel and liquid format and at a concentration of 33% for use as an etchant when restoring teeth using composite filling material. Microscopically, the acid concentration is sufficient to partially dissolve the enamel surface of the tooth so that it is left as an uneven layer with the mineral crystals projecting out. The resin and composite filling material lock onto these projections during the curing process of the restoration, and the resultant filling is secured onto the tooth structure. The etch material is coloured by the manufacturers to ensure that it is clearly visible in case of it accidentally coming into contact with any soft tissues, which would quite easily be burned by this strength of acid.

34 *Correct answer B*: The material's calcium content assists the odontoblasts to form a calcium bridge over the pulp chamber, thereby closing any breaches into the pulp chamber and maintaining the vitality of the tooth. Effectively, this calcium bridge of secondary dentine is the result of the tooth repairing itself after being damaged. As with various other lining materials, calcium hydroxide also helps to chemically calm the pulp and protect it from further chemical irritation, as well as sealing the pulp chamber from residual bacteria.

35 *Correct answer C*: This technique is particularly useful when previous attempts at anaesthetising a tooth have failed, as the intra-osseous technique works immediately and rarely fails. Two small holes are drilled through the cortical plate of bone distal and mesial to the tooth to be anaesthetised, and then a special needle is used to inject the anaesthetic solution directly through the hole and into the cancellous bone of the jaw, immediately around the tooth roots. The lips and cheeks are not affected, and the anaesthetic effect wears off relatively quickly.

36 *Correct answer C*: Chemical waste is not incinerated but disposed of safely in accordance with the chemicals involved. If amalgam were incinerated, poisonous mercury vapour would be released so extracted teeth containing amalgam fillings are placed in tooth pots and disposed of as non-infectious hazardous waste. Although teeth are body parts (which are usually considered as infectious), the risk of mercury poisoning due to incineration is considered higher than the risk of infection in this case. Teeth without amalgam fillings present are placed in the sharps bin and disposed of as infectious waste by incineration.

37 *Correct answer C*: Large composite restorations should therefore be built up in increments, with each one being cured before the addition of the next. Otherwise, the base of a large restoration may remain uncured, and the filling will be unstable and eventually fail.

38 *Correct answer C*: Visible contamination with saliva and blood should be rinsed off the impression before it is inserted into the disinfectant bath; otherwise, the disinfectant solution in the bath will quickly become contaminated with gross debris and require changing. The impression will be rinsed again after removal from the bath, to remove excess disinfectant solution, and then wrapped in damp gauze to prevent drying. Spraying the impression is not a recommended technique of disinfection.

39 *Correct answer B*: Amalgam traps are placed at one of various points within the design of dental suction units, so that all aspirated fluids have to pass through the trap before flowing into the drains. All solid and semi-solid debris (including amalgam waste) is caught in the trap and prevented from entering the drains and therefore the environment. The traps are emptied periodically into the waste amalgam collection container. Amalgam separators are connected to sink drains so that any amalgam debris that has been dislodged from instruments during reprocessing procedures is caught here and prevented from entering the drains.

40 *Correct answer D*: Vasoconstrictors such as adrenaline and felypressin act by constricting and closing any small blood vessels in the area of the injection site. This prevents the circulation from removing the anaesthetic solution from the area until the vessels open again and therefore provides a longer period of action of the anaesthetic. Without a vasoconstrictor in use, the anaesthetic and its numbing effects will wear off in less than twenty minutes in many patients.

41 *Correct answer C*: The release of fluoride from glass ionomer restorations makes them particularly useful in deciduous fillings, where the pulp chambers are much larger and easily breached during cavity preparation. Shallower cavities can be cut, with potentially some caries bacteria still present, but these will be prevented from continuing their attack on the dentine by the fluoride released from the filling material. Composite is also adhesive to etched enamel and is stronger than glass ionomer. Glass ionomers cannot be polished.

42 *Correct answer D*: A class II cavity always involves posterior teeth only and may represent any of the following cavities; a mesio-occlusal, a disto-occlusal, a mesio-disto-occlusal or any of these with an extension onto a side surface of the tooth.

43 *Correct answer A*: The globules are best collected in a syringe and placed directly into the mercury/amalgam waste pot. Bleach has no effect on the release of mercury vapour following a spillage, and the Health and Safety

Executive need only be contacted following a large spillage. Vacuuming the area should never be carried out, as this disperses the dangerous mercury vapour even more widely into the atmosphere.

44 *Correct answer D*: The technique of carrying out a pulpotomy is an attempt to maintain the vitality of a tooth when the root pulp has not been exposed to potential contamination. It is usually carried out in the adult teeth of child patients where an event such as trauma has exposed the coronal pulp only. The young root pulp tissue, especially where the tooth has an open apex, has a good chance of maintaining its vitality and allowing the tooth to continue root formation once the contaminated coronal pulp has been removed and the tooth restored.

45 *Correct answer B*: Alginate impressions must not be allowed to dry out, as they shrink dramatically and become distorted. All three of the other options are impression materials that remain stable and accurate when dry.

46 *Correct answer C*: An inlay is effectively a filling made in a laboratory to seal a cavity, using solid materials such as gold or porcelain rather than the plastic materials used for fillings (amalgam, glass ionomer and so on). The cavity has to be carefully prepared so that its walls have no undercuts; otherwise, the inlay cannot be seated. Conversely, conventional cavities are designed with undercuts to improve the retention of the plastic filling materials.

47 *Correct answer B*: The body attempts to excrete all mercury through the kidneys, but it becomes lodged and trapped in the fine vessels and gradually blocks them, causing permanent kidney damage and ultimately kidney failure. Significant amounts of mercury would need to be inhaled or ingested to damage the lungs or stomach, respectively. Mercury does not tend to cross the blood–brain barrier.

48 *Correct answer D*: The end piece of the archwire is passed through the tube on the molar tooth and clipped off distally using end cutters. The tube can either be cemented directly to the tooth, or it can be soldered onto a molar band, and then the band is cemented onto the tooth.

49 *Correct answer D*: Bone rongeurs are surgical instruments used to nibble away at small pieces of the bone so that a smoother surface is produced, which then allows healing of the overlying mucoperiosteum to occur. Dissecting forceps are used to hold flaps of tissue taut during suturing, and mosquito forceps are correctly used to clamp severed arteries and prevent blood loss during a surgical procedure, although they are often used as needle holders during suturing. The osteotrimmer is used to remove pathological material from bony cavities, such as cysts.

50 *Correct answer C*: A functional appliance is an orthodontic device used to correct jaw malocclusions. All three of the other options are devices used to successfully replace one or more missing teeth.

51 *Correct answer C*: Zinc phosphate cement is adhesive by mechanically locking onto any microscopic irregularities on the surface of the tooth and the inner surface of the fixed prosthesis. All three of the other options are cements that are also chemically adhesive to these surfaces and therefore are overall more adhesive than zinc phosphate. The main advantage of this material is that its setting time can be manipulated to suit the clinician, depending whether a fast or slow set is required.

52 *Correct answer A*: This reacts with the sulphur and water to create a mercury-absorbent paste, which is painted around the spillage to contain it and then over it to cover the spillage. Once dry, the paste and the underlying spillage are wiped up with damp towels and safely disposed of in the correct waste disposal vessel. None of the other three options are materials found in the mercury spillage kit.

53 *Correct answer D*: The administration of an inferior dental nerve block involves the location of the needle tip through various layers of soft tissue and muscle to the mandibular foramen on the inner surface of the ramus of the mandible. A long and wide gauge needle is required to reach this point without bending or snapping. An aspirating technique must be used to avoid injecting into the surrounding blood vessels.

54 *Correct answer A*: Hand files or those designed for use with special endodontic handpieces are inserted into the canals to engage the canal wall, twisted and then scraped against the wall as they are pulled out. This removes a layer of dentine from the inner wall of the canal, along with any pulp or bacterial debris lying there. When the canal is filed systematically in this way, it is both widened and debrided around the natural shape of the canal. Reamers can only be used in a circular action and will fail to contact some areas of the canal walls when an oval shape is present (as many canals are). The two other options are not used for to clean and shape the canal.

55 *Correct answer D*: Immediate replacement dentures are constructed using a model of the patient's teeth, including those the denture will replace. The technician removes these teeth from the model and constructs the denture accordingly. It is fitted at the same appointment as the extraction procedure is carried out, to be inserted immediately into the extraction spaces. A try-in cannot be carried out because the teeth to be extracted would still be present in the patient's mouth.

OUTCOME 4

Understand the Purpose and Stages of Different Dental Procedures

Questions

1 A class II cavity has been prepared for amalgam restoration in an upper molar tooth. Which one of the following items must be used by the operator before the filling can be placed?
   A Articulating paper
   B Gingival retraction cord
   C Matrix outfit
   D Wooden wedge

2 Which one of the following options is a reason for restoring a permanent tooth but not necessarily a deciduous tooth?
   A Aesthetics
   B Alleviate pain
   C Maintain space in the dental arch
   D Restore masticatory function

3 Which one of the following materials may be used to construct a temporary crown but not a permanent crown?
   A Acrylic
   B Ceramic
   C Gold
   D Non-precious metal

Questions and Answers for Diploma in Dental Nursing, Level 3, First Edition. Carole Hollins.
© 2016 John Wiley & Sons, Ltd. Published 2016 by John Wiley & Sons, Ltd.

4 An inlay is a restoration produced in a laboratory to restore a cavity in a tooth, unlike a filling that is produced at the chair side. Which of the following techniques will be used during the filling procedure, but not during the inlay procedure?

A Use of anaesthetic

B Use of dentinal pins

C Use of lining

D Use of undercuts

5 During denture construction, the patient will attend for a trial insertion of the dentures with the teeth set in wax rims. Which one of the following instruments is used for fine wax adjustments at this stage?

A Articulator

B Le Cron carver

C Plaster knife

D Wax knife

6 Which one of the following terms describes an appliance used to close an anatomical defect of the oral cavity that has been left following surgery, such as following the removal of an oral cancer lesion?

A Functional appliance

B Immediate denture

C Obturator

D Overdenture

7 Which one of the following techniques is most likely to be carried out to save a tooth from extraction when the patient is suffering from irreversible pulpitis?

A Apicectomy

B Pulp capping

C Pulpectomy

D Pulpotomy

8 Cavity preparation in permanent teeth is often slightly different to that carried out in deciduous teeth. Which one of the following may occur during cavity preparation in a deciduous tooth only?

A Administration of local anaesthetic

B Incomplete removal of deep caries

C Use of a temporary filling material

D Use of glass ionomer

9 An inlay is a fixed prosthodontic restoration used to restore a cavity in a tooth. Which one of the following materials is not suitable for inlay construction?

A Ceramic

B Composite

C Glass ionomer

D Gold

10 Which one of the following is the usual retentive component present on a removable orthodontic appliance?

   A Adams crib
   B Band
   C Canine retractor
   D Finger spring

11 Which one of the following treatment procedures is not carried out for deciduous teeth?

   A Crown placement
   B Extraction
   C Filling
   D Pulpectomy

12 Which one of the following options is the most likely reason for a patient to be provided with a veneer?

   A Improve the bite
   B Mask discolouration
   C Replace a missing tooth
   D Strengthen a tooth

13 Which one of the following materials is not used to cement a molar band to a tooth as part of a fixed orthodontic appliance?

   A Composite filler
   B Glass ionomer
   C Zinc phosphate
   D Zinc polycarboxylate

14 Missing teeth can be replaced by various dental techniques, such as dentures and bridges. Which one of the following is the term used to describe the branch of dentistry concerned with the replacement of missing teeth?

   A Gerodontics
   B Orthodontics
   C Paedodontics
   D Prosthodontics

15 What is the main benefit to the patient of having a missing tooth replaced by an implant rather than a bridge?

   A Better aesthetics
   B Cost of treatment
   C Permanent tooth replacement
   D Single tooth involvement

16 A tooth may require one of several types of endodontic treatment to avoid extraction. Which type of treatment involves the use of endodontic files during its completion?

   A Apicectomy

   B Pulp capping

   C Pulpectomy

   D Pulpotomy

17 Which one of the following actions is usually achieved with the use of a fixed orthodontic appliance rather than with a removable orthodontic appliance?

   A Correction of crossbite

   B Derotation of teeth

   C Reduction of overbite

   D Reduction of overjet

18 After a tooth has been extracted, a patient may be fitted with a temporary bridge. What is the main reason for a temporary rather than a permanent bridge to be fitted in this case?

   A Allow bone resorption to occur

   B Allow patient to get used to a bridge

   C Lower cost of temporary bridge

   D Provide correct occlusion

19 Partial denture construction is usually completed in several stages. Which one of the following stages may be omitted when constructing a denture to replace a single tooth?

   A Bite recording

   B Fitting

   C Initial impression

   D Try-in

20 Missing teeth may be replaced by dentures, bridges or implants. Which one of the following options is the main reason for a denture to fail in its intended purpose of successful tooth replacement?

   A Easily fractured

   B Easily removed

   C Too difficult to clean

   D Too expensive

21 Which one of the following is the term used to correctly describe the method of bony retention achieved to hold an implant in place in the jaw bone?

   A Adhesion

   B Alveoplasty

   C Conditioning

   D Osseointegration

22 Which one of the following treatment aims can be achieved using either a functional or fixed orthodontic appliance, but not by using a removable appliance?

A Correction of crossbite

B Correction of jaw relationship

C Correction of tooth position in arch

D Reduction of overjet

23 Which one of the following statements is false in relation to the aftercare advice given to a patient who has recently been fitted with a chrome-cobalt partial denture?

A Clean the denture over a filled sink to avoid fracture

B Remove the denture from the mouth to clean it

C Use bleach-based soaking agents to disinfect the denture

D Wear the denture every day

24 A permanent tooth is undergoing restoration by filling. Which one of the following options is the correct sequence of events in this procedure?

A Caries removal, lining, filling and shaping

B Caries removal, shaping, lining and filling

C Shaping, caries removal, lining and filling

D Shaping, lining, caries removal and filling

25 Which one of the following options listed is the main reason for providing a patient with a temporary crown on a root-filled molar tooth?

A Aesthetics

B Maintain occlusion

C Prevent sensitivity

D Strengthen the tooth

Answers

1 *Correct answer C*: Siqveland and Tofflemire matrix outfits are available for use in this situation to enclose the cavity and prevent material spillage into the interproximal region during packing. The outfit must be securely in place around the tooth before beginning to fill the cavity. A wooden wedge may be placed after the matrix outfit to ensure the band is adapted closely to the tooth in the interproximal region. Retraction cord is used during fixed prosthetic preparation procedures, and articulating paper is used after the filling has been placed to ensure there are no premature contacts.

2 *Correct answer A*: As the deciduous teeth are shed naturally between the ages of 6 and 13 years, the aesthetics is of far less importance than it is with permanent teeth. Both dentitions should be restored for all of the three other options.

3 *Correct answer A*: Temporary crowns are in place for a matter of weeks before removal, so they must be easily constructed at the chair side using an inexpensive material, such as acrylic. All three of the other options are materials commonly used to construct permanent crowns.

4 *Correct answer D*: Inlays must be placed in cavities designed with near-parallel sides, with the top of the cavity fractionally wider than the base so that the inlay can be fully seated. If undercuts are present, the inlay will have been constructed with too wide a base and it will be impossible to seat it in the cavity. All three of the other options may be required during both a filling procedure and an inlay procedure.

5 *Correct answer B*: This is a fine knife used for precise wax adjustments at the try-in stage. It can be used to fine trim the wax around the tooth margins or remove shavings of wax from the flanges of the try-in. The wax knife is a more bulky bladed instrument that is used for gross alterations at both the bite registration and the try-in stages. It is usually heated in a flame to assist wax removal. The two other options are not required at the try-in stage of denture construction.

6 *Correct answer C*: The obturator appliance design will extend to completely seal any anatomical defect present. It is made in a similar way to an acrylic denture, with the impression material having to be inserted into the anatomical defect to record it, as well as into the oral cavity to record the dental arches in the usual way. An overdenture is one designed to sit over one or more retained roots.

7 *Correct answer C*: Pulpectomy involves the removal of all pulp tissue from a tooth and is the correct term for conventional root canal therapy/treatment. It is undertaken as the only treatment able to save a tooth from extraction when irreversible pulpitis has developed. Apicectomy is the surgical amputation of the root apex and removal of any associated pathology, while pulp capping is the technique used to sterilise and seal a pinpoint exposure of the coronal pulp. Pulpotomy is the procedure where the contents of the coronal pulp chamber are removed, leaving the radicular pulp intact and usually carried out in newly erupted permanent teeth in children.

8 *Correct answer B*: The pulp chamber of a deciduous tooth is larger and therefore closer to the surface of the tooth than that of a permanent tooth. An accidental exposure is therefore much more likely in deciduous teeth while trying to remove deep caries. As the deciduous teeth are naturally shed, it is acceptable to leave some deep caries in a cavity in these situations. The cavity can be disinfected with medicaments such as cresophene and then restored in the hope that the tooth will remain pain-free and functional until it is naturally exfoliated.

9 *Correct answer C*: The purpose of placing an inlay is to restore a tooth with a stronger material than those used for conventional fillings. While especially hardened composite materials are available for this purpose, there is no glass ionomer equivalent. The composite inlay is constructed in the laboratory as an indirect restoration, in the same way that both ceramic and gold inlays are manufactured.

10 *Correct answer A*: Adams cribs are designed to fit around the molar or premolar teeth and can be tightened using pliers so that they grip the natural undercuts of these teeth and hold the appliance in place. A band is a retentive component of a fixed orthodontic appliance, while a canine retractor and a finger spring are active components of a removable appliance.

11 *Correct answer D*: Full removal of the pulp chamber contents and replacement with gutta-percha to seal the chamber (root canal treatment) is not carried out on deciduous teeth for several reasons. Firstly, the instrumentation and root filling procedure may damage the permanent tooth successor that is developing immediately beneath the deciduous tooth, and secondly, as root resorption occurs before the deciduous tooth is shed, the gutta-percha material will be left behind and may damage the permanent tooth as it tries to erupt or even prevent it from doing so. All three of the other options are procedures that may be carried out on deciduous teeth – pre-formed metal crowns are used posteriorly to conserve these teeth before exfoliation.

12 *Correct answer B*: Veneers tend to be used for aesthetic reasons and especially for masking the discolouration that may develop following root canal treatment. Alternatively, internal tooth bleaching may be used to improve the aesthetics of the tooth. Where the tooth colour is naturally dark, external tooth whitening may be carried out on all of the teeth to improve their appearance. Veneers do not improve the bite of a tooth, as they are just cemented to the labial surface. They also cannot strengthen a tooth nor replace a missing tooth.

13 *Correct answer A*: Conventional composite filling material is not suitable as a luting cement, which would be its function in this situation, as it is too stiff to apply easily and too adhesive to be completely removed from the enamel during the debonding of the fixed appliance at the end of the treatment. However, special flowable composite materials may be used for this purpose, as may all three of the other options listed.

14 *Correct answer D*: This branch of dentistry involves both fixed and removable devices used to restore teeth and replace them. Gerodontics is concerned with the treatment of elderly patients and their teeth, while paedodontics is the branch of dentistry concerned with the dental treatment of children. Orthodontics is the branch of dentistry concerned with the treatment of malocclusions.

15 *Correct answer D*: An implant is a titanium post screwed into the alveolar bone, which then has a crown placed on the top to replace a missing tooth. No other teeth are involved in the implant procedure. However, a bridge involves attachments to one or more other teeth that are joined to the false tooth replacing the missing one, so one or more adjacent teeth will need preparing to hold the bridge in place. Adhesive bridges require minimal tooth preparation but can be dislodged if the patient has a heavy bite, so they cannot be used in many situations.

16 *Correct answer C*: Hand files are engine-driven files used during the pulpectomy procedure to clean and shape the root canal before the root filling is placed. They are not used in any of the three other endodontic procedures listed.

17 *Correct answer B*: Tooth derotation is the most difficult movement to achieve and involves some considerable force being applied to the tooth during the process. This force is usually sufficient to dislodge a removable appliance, so that the energy required to move the tooth is lost. As the fixed appliance is cemented to all of the teeth, greater constant forces can be applied and tooth derotation is normally achieved after several months. Removable appliances can be used to achieve all three of the other actions listed.

18 *Correct answer A*: Once a tooth has been extracted, the alveolar bone surrounding its socket undergoes a period of resorption and remodelling, which can take up to 6 months to complete. During this time, the ridge shape will alter and shrink, often leaving visible gaps beneath the temporary bridge. If the permanent bridge had been placed immediately, it would eventually require removal and remake so that the resorption gaps are accommodated in the new design. A far better technique is to fit a temporary bridge for this period and then replace it with a well-fitting permanent bridge when resorption has ceased.

19 *Correct answer A*: With a full complement of teeth otherwise, the technician will be able to locate the models in the correct occlusion without having to record the bite first. All three of the other stages are required to be carried out to ensure that the design, shade, tooth mould and fit of the appliance are correct.

20 *Correct answer B*: Dentures are the only devices used to replace missing teeth that can be removed by the patient – bridges are permanently cemented to their teeth, and implants are permanently integrated into their jaw bone. The wearing of the denture is under the control of the patient, and the success of the device therefore depends entirely on their compliance with the wearing instructions given by the dental team. Dentures replacing posterior teeth only are especially likely to fail, as they are not required for aesthetics and many patients do not appreciate the importance of easing the occlusal load on their remaining teeth by wearing the denture.

21 *Correct answer D*: Once inserted into the socket and initially screwed into place, the local alveolar bone grows into and around the structure of the implant so that it becomes incorporated into the bone tissue – this is called osseointegration.

22 *Correct answer B*: A class II malocclusion exists where the lower jaw is behind its correct position in relation to the upper jaw, and this can be corrected using a functional appliance or a fixed appliance, but not a removable appliance. The functional technique uses the muscular forces of the jaw during growth to gradually reposition the lower jaw into its correct position. The fixed technique uses elastics running from the upper canines to the lower first molars to achieve the same result. Elastics can be used in the opposite way to correct class III malocclusions too. A removable appliance is worn in one arch only and therefore cannot be used to correct jaw relationships.

23 *Correct answer C*: Bleach-based denture soaking products will gradually corrode the structure of the metal, discolouring it with an unsightly black tarnish and causing pitting of the metal surface. All three of the other options apply to all dentures, including chrome-cobalt designs.

24 *Correct answer B*: All caries must be removed from the cavity before any other stage can be carried out. This procedure may have automatically produced a retentive shape for the filling, but if not, then the cavity must be correctly shaped so that the filling is not easily dislodged. The base can then be lined to protect the underlying pulp, and then the cavity is filled.

25 *Correct answer B*: Once the tooth has been prepared for the crown, it has effectively been removed from the normal occlusion – this is how space is created to fit the crown without altering the patient's bite. If a temporary crown is not placed, the tooth will gradually erupt slightly until it comes into contact with the opposing tooth so that they bite together again – but the space has then been lost for the crown to be fitted. So the temporary crown is placed to maintain the correct occlusion. A posterior tooth is not usually visible and therefore aesthetics are not an issue. A root-filled tooth is dead and will not suffer from sensitivity if left uncovered while the permanent crown is made. The materials used in temporary crowns are not strong.

Index

Page numbers in **bold** refer to pages having answers to the questions

---

Questions and Answers for Diploma in Dental Nursing, Level 3, First Edition. Carole Hollins.
© 2016 John Wiley & Sons, Ltd. Published 2016 by John Wiley & Sons, Ltd.